AF555918

Zoonotic Parasites of Livestock
Diagnosis and Contol

Zoonotic Parasites of Livestock
Diagnosis and Contol

Mohd Rashid
Rajesh Katoch
Mudasir Sultana
Kafil Hussain
H.K.Sharma

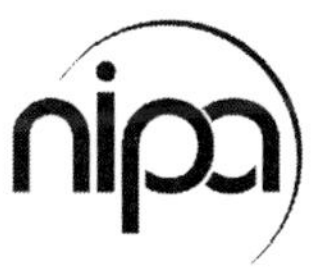

NEW INDIA PUBLISHING AGENCY
New Delhi – 110 034

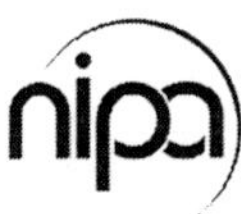

NEW INDIA PUBLISHING AGENCY
101, Vikas Surya Plaza, CU Block, LSC Market
Pitam Pura, New Delhi 110 034, India
Phone: + 91 (11)27 34 17 17 Fax: + 91(11) 27 34 16 16
Email: info@nipabooks.com
Web: www.nipabooks.com

Feedback at feedbacks@nipabooks.com

ISBN 978-93-86546-81-4

Composed and Designed by NIPA

Preface

The state of Jammu & Kashmir is an agrarian state and about 80% of population is associated with livestock farming. This sector plays an important role in socioeconomic upliftment of rural community. This manual has been prepared by the Principle Investigator NRDMS/DST-project with the support of senior Faculty members. It will be used as a tool of interventional strategies for prevention and control of parasitic zoonoses of livestock and their rearers belonging to socio-economically poor communities by imparting knowledge through training of field veterinarians. It will be useful as a conceptual guide as well as reference material for trainers. Moreover, some part of it could be used as reading material for participants. The various aspects of livestock farming, management, disease diagnoses and prevention and control measures have been included into the training manual. Livestock rearing are popular because of the prolificacy, less investment and minimal skills that are needed for success. In addition, state is an agrarian and livestock farming play an important role in livelihood of rural people. However, the present manual focuses on some modern technological aspects of disease diagnoses, measures for prevention and control, care and management of livestock for enhancing the productivity.

Simple changes in care and management of livestock can significantly improve production and the living conditions of many rural families in terms of enhanced nutrition and income generation through the sale of animal and their products. Improved animal production, early disease diagnoses, adoption of simple measures for care and management are therefore a low-cost and important aspect of rural development.

This manual aims to provide, for Veterinary Doctors, modern practices on the production of dairy animal, sheep and goat farming to know how productivity can be improved by introducing appropriate, low- cost approaches. The manual describes the steps that can be taken to improve health of animals and reduce the mortality. More costly techniques such as supplementary feeding, intensive rearing are also covered in this manual. This information could be used for planning, implementing and monitoring livestock programme. It is expected that service providers will educate the farmers about the extra costs and labour that would be required for more intensive livestock farming.

Editors

Aims of Training

The aim of this training book is to update the knowledge of field functionaries, such as veterinarians, laboratory technicians in identifying the important parasites of economic and public health significance of livestock. This training manual will provide a bench mark aids in diagnosing intestinal infections from faecal samples. To update the knowledge of field veterinarians lectures on important aspects have been included in the manual which will be discussed in due course of time by the experts from the faculty.

At the end of the training course the learners should be able to perform the following laboratory techniques:

- Specific laboratory techniques
- Direct microscopic examination of smears
- Collection and preservation of samples and parasites
- Concentration of eggs for quantitative analysis
- Staining techniques of intestinal protozoa
- Identification of parasites up to genus and species
- Quantification of eggs.

Title of Training: Diagnosis and control of zoonotic parasites of livestock and their rearers through management, planning and socio mobilization.

Training Objective: At the end of the training program the participants will be able to :

1. Update knowledge and skill on livestock farming.
2. Analyze the possible interventions to improve the livestock development scenario by control of parasitic zoonoses.
3. Assess possible losses a farmer incurs due to various management problems and its remedial measures.
4. Explore possible ways to motivate the farmers for adopting modern technology.
5. Find out the prevalence of zoonotic parasitic diseases of the area.

6. Analyze the community mobilization techniques suitable for dairy and small animal rearers.

Time Table

Day 1	Inauguration Introduction of the Programme	Present status of livestock in J&K and its role in socio- economy of farmers	Community and its diversity	Group approach
Day 2	Participatory Project Planning	Problem identification in Sheep, Goat and Cattle, Buffaloes rearing to enhance income.	Action Planning	Care and management of dairy animals
Day 3	Common zoonotic Diseases of Sheep and Goat and their prevention & control	Common external parasitic infestation in livestock and their control	Common external parasitic infestation in livestock and their control	Care and management of Sheep and Goat
Day 4	Preparation of Small Scale Sheep, Goat project & their economic analysis	Action plan of Sheep and Goat Development	Group discussion	Practical
Day 5	Development of comprehensive plan potentiality and intervention	Presentation of the final comprehensive Action Plan.	Practical	Valediction & Feedback

List of zoonotic parasites to Discussed in the Programme

1. Cryptosporidium parvum
2. Entmoeba histolytica
3. Giardia lamblia
4. Toxoplasma gondii.
5. Ancylostoma caninum
6. Bunostomum
7. Echinococcus (Hydatid cyst)
8. Faciola hepatica
9. Strongyloides
10. Strongyles
11. Toxocara species
12. Mites

Contents

1

An Overview of Helminthes of Zoonotic and Public Health Importance

M. Rashid and Alveena Ganai
Faculty of Veterinary Sciences & Animal Husbandry, SKUAST-Jammu-181102

Helminths include the nematodes (roundworms), trematodes (flukes) and the cestodes (tapeworms). The adult worms live in intestine and discharge the eggs or larvae that comes out with the faeces. Therefore, diagnosis is based on the detection of eggs or larvae in faecal samples.

Overview of Nematode infections in humans and animals

The phylum Nematoda, (roundworms), is the second largest phylum in the animal kingdom, encompassing up to 500,000 species. Members of Nematoda are elongated, with bilaterally symmetric bodies that contain an intestinal system and a large body cavity. According to a report approximately 60 species of roundworms parasitize humans. Intestinal roundworm infections constitute the largest group of helminthic diseases in humans. According to 2005 report of World Health Organization (WHO), approximately 0.807-1.221 billion humans suffers from ascariasis, 604-795 million from trichuriasis and 576-740 million from hookworm infections worldwide.

Ascariasis

Ascaris lumbricoides infect 0.807-1.3 billion people worldwide with 250 million associated in causing morbidity. In contrast, the closely related species *Ascaris suum* and *Trichuris suis* in pigs have global distribution, with infected pigs found in most production systems. In areas where pigs and humans live in close proximity or where pig manure is used as fertilizer for growing vegetables for human consumption, there is a potential risk of cross infections.

Each species has its specific ascarid, *A. vitulorun* in cattle, *A. equorum* in horses, *A. suum* in pigs and *A. lumbricoides* in man. The worms found in man and pigs are morphologically and serologically indistinguish-able, but are apparently of "physiological" or "host" varieties. In all animal species, young ones are seriously affected. In pigs up to 4-5 months of age the important clinical signs are poor growth and susceptible to other diseases due to poor resistance. Enzootic pneumonia of pigs and swine influenza becomes very serious when accompa-nied by ascariasis. Adult worms may be vomitted up and occasional cases of obstructive jaundice and intestinal obstruction or rupture occur. Similar symptoms are also observed in calves and foals. In adult animals, no clinical symptoms are observed.

Trichuriasis

Trichuris spp infections are common in young calves and yearlings, and children, worldwide. The eggs are resistant and infections are likely to persist on infective premises. Clinical signs are not clearly observed, but occasionally in heavy infections, dark faeces, anemia and anorexia have been seen.

There is a worldwide distribution of *Trichuris trichiura* in humans, with an estimated 1 billion human infections in Asia. Within the United States 2.2 million people are thought to be infected. Poor hygiene is associated with trichuriasis as well as the consumption of shaded moist soil, or food that may have been fecally contaminated. Children are especially vulnerable to infection due to their high exposure risk. Eggs are infective about 2–3 weeks after they are deposited in the soil under favourable conditions of warmth and moisture in tropical areas.

Infection occurs through ingestion of eggs and is more common in tropical areas. Whipworms eggs are passed in the faeces of infected persons/animals, and if an infected human faeces or animal dung used as fertilizer, eggs are deposited on soil where they can mature into an infective stage. Ingestion of these eggs "can happen when hands or fingers that have contaminated dirt on them are put in the mouth or by consuming vegetables or fruits that have not been carefully cooked, washed or peeled." The eggs hatch in the small intestine and then move into the wall of the small intestine and develop. On reaching adulthood, the thinner end (the front of the worm) burrows into the large intestine and the thicker end hangs into the lumen and mates with nearby worms. The females can grow to 50 mm (2.0 μm) long. Neither the male nor the female has much of a visible tail past the anus.

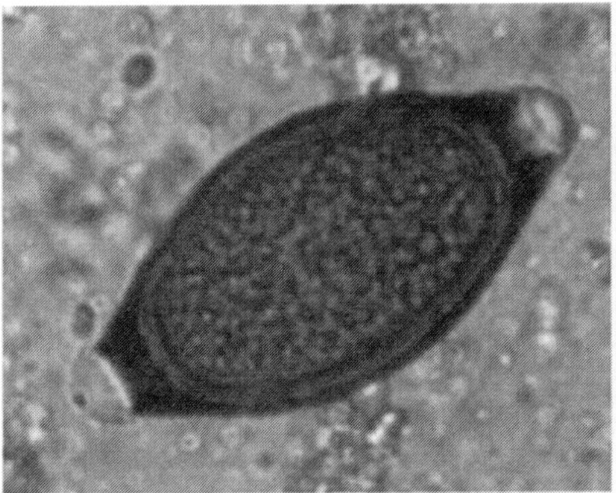

Trichuris ovis

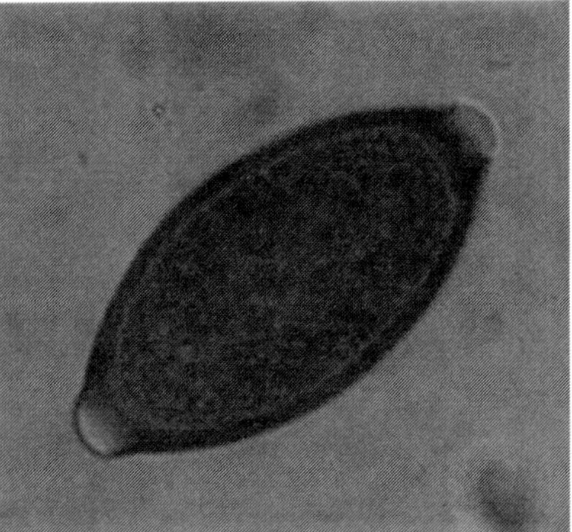

Trichuris vulpis

Ancylostomiasis and Uncinariasis

Hookworms

The larvae of *Ancylostoma caninum, Ancylostoma braziliense, Ancylostoma duodenale* and *Uncinaria stenocephala* get entry through the skin and may give rise to a marked local reaction in the skin and subcutis. These worms occur in the small intestines of dog, cat, fox and man. Hookworms infect over 1.25 billion people throughout the world. The hookworms (*Necator americanus, Ancylostoma duodenale*) are medically important human parasites and cause serious morbidity in many parts of the world. The adult worms are small and live in the small intestine. They measure about 1.0 to 1.5 cm in length. Although the adult worms of these two species are easily identified on the basis of presence of cutting plates (*N. americanus*) or teeth (*A. duodenale*) around the mouth, the eggs they produce are nearly identical. The typical hookworm egg measures 60-75 μm by 36-40 μm. It has a clear, thin shell and the ovum is usually in the 4 or 8 cell stage or sometimes more advanced.

The adult pararites attach themselves to the mucosa of the intestine and suck blood. They inject into the wounds the secreting of their cephalic glands which prevent coagulation. The blood-sucking action of the parasites cause severe anaemia and deplete the body of iron, thus preventing further formation of Erythrocytes.

Cutaneous larva migrans (abbreviated **CLM**) is a skin disease in humans, caused by the larvae of various nematode parasites of the hookworm family (Ancylostomatidae). The most common species causing this disease are *Ancylostoma caninum, Ancylostoma braziliense, Ancylostoma duodenale*. These parasites live in the intestines of dogs, cats, and wild animals and should not be confused with other members of the hookworm family for which humans are definitive hosts, namely *Ancylostoma duodenale* and *Necator americanus*.

Colloquially called **creeping eruption** due to its presentation, the disease is also somewhat ambiguously known as "**ground itch**" or (in some parts of the Southern USA) "**sandworms**", as the larvae like to live in sandy soil. Another vernacular name is **plumber's itch**. The medical term CLM literally means "wandering larvae in the skin".

Creeping eruption occurs in man and is characterised by the presence of progressively developing thickened tracks in the skin accompanied by itching. It is caused by wandering larvae of *Ancylostoma braziliense* and *Uncinaria stenocephala* but the most frequent cause is the larvae of *A. braziliense*.

It occurs chiefly on the feet, legs and gluteal region of children and is seen mostly in warm climates, where moist and sandy soil is found. Thus, dog and cats may be infected by children, and vice versa.

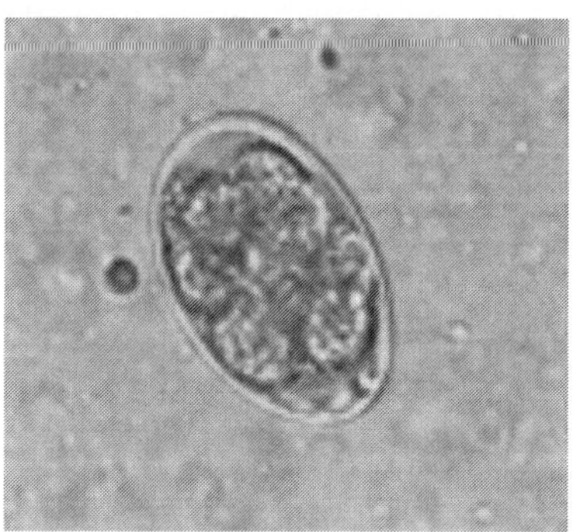

Ancylostoma caninum

Visceral larva migrans

Visceral larva migrans is a condition caused by the migratory larvae of certain nematodes in humans and first reported by Beaver, et al. (1952). Humans' beings are dead-end host. Nematodes causing such zoonotic infections are *Toxocara canis, Toxocara cati* and *Ascaris suum*. These nematodes can infect but not mature in humans and after migrating through the intestinal wall, travel with the blood stream to various organs where they cause inflammation and damage. Affected organs can include the liver, heart (causing myocarditis) and the CNS (causing dysfunction, seizures, and coma). A special variant is ocular larva migrans where usually *T. canis* larvae travel to the eye.

Only a few roundworm eggs are necessary to cause larva migrans in the human child or adult. However, visceral larva migrans seems to affect children aged 1–4 more often while ocular larva migrans more frequently affects children aged 7–8. Between 4.6% and 23% of U.S. children have been infected with the dog roundworm egg. This number is much higher in other parts of the world, such as Colombia, where up to 81% of children have been infected (Artem Cheprasov, 2012).

Trichostrongylosis

Trichostrongylosis is caused by more than 30 species. Most of them are parasites of herbivores, but 10 species have been reported infecting humans. Out of them *T. colubriformis* is an important zoonotic species found infecting man and goats in a village of Loas Angel. *Trichostrongylus* species occurs throughout the world mostly as animal parasites. However, humans become infected with *Trichostrongylus* species mainly by ingesting infective-stage larvae or infrequently penetrating to the skin. Species of *Trichostrongylus* are usually small worms, less than 1 cm in length that live in the small intestine. Trichostrongyle eggs resemble the eggs of the hookworms but are larger in size, 70-95 μm by 40-50 μm. Thus, detailed discrimination of *Trichostrongylus* spp. is important for efficient prevention and control programs of the parasite.

Strongyloidiasis

Strongyloides spp. infect a range of domestic animal species worldwide. In general, there is host specificity for each *strongyloides* spp.

However, this has been based primarily on morphology and not genetic confirmation. In studies on the prevalence and impact of infection, it is generally assumed that the species present is the one that has been previously identified as belonging to that host. Despite being capable of infecting different age groups, clinical disease is most often encountered in the young animals. In herbivores, the small, oval, thin-shelled, larvated (atypical) eggs are easily recognized when faecal material is subject to flotation, a diagnostic procedure commonly used.

Strongyloides stercoralis

This is an important nematode parasite of humans having ability of autoinfection and dissemination throughout the organ systems of immunocompromized or immunosuppressed individuals or others with malignancies, e.g. lymphoma. This nematode parasite produces rhabditoid larvae instead of eggs, which are found in faeces. The larva measures 180-380 μm in length by 14–20 μm in diameter. It has a short buccal capsule, a slender, pointed tail and a prominent genital primordium. The larva could easily be recognized, by staining with iodine.

Overview of Trematodes

The trematodes are usually referred as flukes. They are solid-bodied worms, hermaphroditic (except schistosomes) and have a complicated life cycle that always involves a snail as intermediate host and in many instances, a second intermediate host. Depending on the species, trematodes inhabit the intestine, liver, lungs or blood vessels of their hosts.

Schistosoma species

The schistosomes cause the most important trematode infections. They infect over 200 million people. These worms live in the small blood vessels associated with the liver, intestine and bladder (depending on the species) and cause extreme pathology, morbidity and mortality in individuals with heavy, chronic infections. They have a snail intermediate host and transmission is water-related. All of the schistosome species produce non-operculated eggs which are passed in faeces or urine (depending on the species), and each egg has a spine on some part of the shell.

Schistosoma japonicum is transmitted in Asia. The egg which is found in faeces measures 70-100 μm by 55-65 μm, has a thin shell with an often inconspicuous, small lateral spine. The egg contains a miracidium. The shell is sticky, causing debris to adhere to the surface and making it more difficult to identify.

Foodborne Trematodes

There are a number of species of foodborne trematodes or flukes that live in the liver and produce operculate eggs that are shed in faeces.

Clonorchis sinensis is transmitted in Asia. The parasite is easily recognized by its small egg that measures 27-35 μm by 12-19 μm. The operculum is seated on a prominent rim or shoulder.

At the opposite pole there may be a small protuberance. The egg contains a miracidium.

The related liver fluke, ***Opisthorchis viverrini,*** is transmitted in Southeast Asia and parts of Europe and produces an egg almost indistinguishable from that of *C. sinensis.*

Fasciola hepatica

This liver fluke is transmitted throughout the world, especially in sheep-raising countries. The adult fluke is large (about 3 cm), lives in the biliary ducts and produces eggs which are passed in faeces as coloured eggs.

The egg is large, measuring 130-150 μm by 63-90 μm, has a thin shell that is brown in colour, a small operculum and is unembryonated when passed in faeces.

The related intestinal fluke, ***Fasciolopsis buski,*** occurs in Asia has an egg almost indistinguishable from that of *F. hepatica*. The *F. buski* egg lacks the thickening at the abopercular end of the shell characteristic of *F. hepatica*.

Paragonimus westermani

Paragonimiasis occurs in Asia, Africa and the western hemisphere. The adult worms are encapsulated in the tissues of the lungs and eggs are discharged in sputum and in faeces. The egg is moderately large, ovoid in shape, has a thick, brown shell and prominent operculum. It is unembryonated when found in sputum or faeces. They have the size of 80-120 µm by 45-70 µm. Other species of *Paragonimus* infect people in various parts of the world. The eggs are all very similar in appearance but differ in size.

Overview of Cestodes

The adult cestodes live in the human intestine and those of interest here produce eggs which are found in faeces.

Taenia solium and *Taenia saginata*

The adults parasite live in the intestine and produces eggs there. They are very large worms, several meters in length. Proglottids as well as eggs appear in faeces. The eggs of the two species are identical they are round to oval in shape, measuring 35-43 µm in diameter and have a thick, radially-striated shell. The egg contains 6-hooked embryo called an oncosphere. These eggs must be handled with extreme care because the egg of *Taenia solium* is infective to humans and produces cysticercosis.

Hymenolepiasis

Hymenolepis worms live in the intestines of rats and are common in warm climates, and are generally found in the faeces of rats, which are consumed by their secondary hosts - beetles. The worms mature into a life form referred to as a "cysticercoid" in the insect; in *H. nana,* the insect is always a beetle. The egg is unique in its appearance. It is small, measuring a size of 30-47 µm in diameter with a thin, colourless shell. The membrane surrounding the hexacanth embryo has 4-8 filaments arising from each pole that fill much of the space between the embryo and the shell. Humans and other animals become infected when they intentionally or unintentionally eat material contaminated by insects. In an infected person, it is possible for the worm's entire lifecycle to be completed in the bowel, so infection can persist for years if left untreated. *H. nana* infections are much more common than *H. diminuta* infections in humans because, in addition to being spread by insects, the disease can be spread directly from person to person by eggs in faeces. When this happens, *H. nana* oncosphere larvae encyst in the intestinal wall and develop into cysticercoids and then adults. These infections were previously common in the southeastern USA, and have been described in crowded environments and individuals confined to institutions. The disease occurs worldwide and *H. nana* eggs can hatch and develop leaving the definitive host unlike most of the tapeworms.

Hymenolepis diminuta

This tapeworm is a natural parasite of rats but also infects humans, especially children. The adult parasite measures up to 60 cm in length, produces eggs which pass in faeces. The egg, which resembles that of *Hymenolepis nana,* is larger measuring 70-85 µm by 60-80 µm and contains a hexacanth embryo. The shell is thick and usually brown in colour. There are no polar filaments emanating from the surface of the hexacanth embryo.

Diphyllobothrium latum

This tapeworm lives in the intestine, measures several meters in length and is found in temperate climates. Its egg is passed in faeces. The egg of *Diphyllobothrium latum* differs from other tapeworms in that it has an operculum. It is ovoid in shape, measures 58-75 µm by 45-50 µm and is unembryonated when found in faeces. There is a small knob on the abopercular end. Sometimes this egg is confused with that of *Paragonimus* spp.

Overview of Protozoa

Giardiasis

Giardiasis is one of the most common intestinal parasitic disease worldwide with an estimated 28,00,000 infections per year in human

(Ali Syed, 2003). *G.duodenalis* is the zoonotic species which can be transmitted from livestock to man and vice versa. It causes self limiting clinical illness characterized by diarrhea, abdominal cramps, bloating, weight loss, malabsorption in man, which usually disappears within few months. Asymptomatic form is more prominent in animals compared to subclinical form in humans, with an infection rate varying from 8% to 30% in children in Asian countries (Feng and Xiao, 2011) and in cattle, prevalence ranges from 2.2% to 50.7% worldwide (Huang *et al.*, 2014). It is endemic throughout the world, may take an epidemic form too. Due to high prevalence disease has public health importance. It is a disease which is associated with insufficient unhygienic water with insanitary conditions prevailing near drinking water sources or use of raw human and animal dung in growing of vegetables etc.

Cryptosporidiosis

Cryptosporidium is a unicellular microscopic intracellular protozoan parasite that infect the microvillus border of the gastrointestinal epithelium as well as respiratory tract of animals and humans. This parasite completes its entire life cycle within a single host. The common feature in this species is the presence of four naked sporozoites, which are contained within a thick walled oocyst without sporocysts. Transmission is mainly by ingestion of sporulated oocysts through contaminated feed and water. Cross infection occurs between domestic and laboratory animals and man. A wide variety of domestic and wild animals serve as a source of human infection, causing significant morbidity and mortality, which now represents the third major cause of diarrheal disease worldwide. Various studies have revealed that cattle, pigs and wild rodents as important reservoirs of parasite *Cryptosporidium* with the prevalence of 11.32% to 69.32% in India (Bhat *et al.*, 2012) and 27.25% in Jammu region (Ganai, 2015). Cryptosporidiosis in livestock has been reported from different parts of the world with approximately 45.5% in USA, 24.5% in UK, 26% in USSR, 40% in Germany and 27% in Hungary (Bhat *et al.*, 2012). Till date about 25 species of *Cryptosporidium* have been reported based on host specificity and among them the most commonly encountered *Cryptosporidium* species in livestock are *C. parvum*, *C. andersoni*, *C. bovis* and *C. ryanae* (formerly known as deer like genotype). The species *Cryptosporidium parvum* may have the most complex epidemiology between them all because of its capacity to infect humans through zoonotic and anthroponotic transmission. *Cryptosporidium parvum* causes scour in young, unweaned young animals, but weaned and adult animals can also be infected. Weaned and adult animals normally do not exhibit signs of disease, but excrete oocysts that may contaminate the environment.

Cryptosporidium andersoni affects the digestive glands of the abomasums of older calves and adult cattle. Some infected animals exhibit reduced weight gain, but do not develop diarrhea. Cryptosporidium bovis and C. ryanae have been described recently. *Cryptosporidium bovis* is a highly prevalent species that infects primarily past-weaned calves. Infected young animals can exhibit clinical signs ranging from asymptomatic infection to profuse diarrhea and dehydration. These animals contaminate their immediate environment, as total oocysts output per infected calf can be upto 10^{10} over a week.

Among the entire animals hosts young animals are the most important from public health point of view, as they may serve as a source of human infection through faecal-oral route. In industrialized countries, epidemic cryptosporidiosis can occur in adult by food borne and water borne sources and the extreme robustness of the oocyst, the infective stage of *Cryptosporidium* parasite, accounts for the importance of indirect transmission through ingestion of contaminated water and food.

Cryptosporidiosis is a major public health problem both in developing and developed countries. The disease is characterised by acute gastrointestinal disturbances, heamorrhagic or mucoid diarrhea, fever, lethargy, anorexia, malnutrition, loss of condition and stunted growth. A major problem concerning cryptosporidiosis is the lack of an effective means for prevention and therapy of this disease. The oocysts is the infective stage of *Cryptosporidium* that is exceptionally resistant to environmental stress and harsh chemical treatments, which allows the parasites to stably persist outside a host. Clinically asymptomatic animals continuously shed oocysts, contaminating the environment and serves as a source of human infection. The increasing population of animals and water borne Cryptosporidiosis outbreaks have placed a great threat to the community and require special attention on the pathogen and disease mechanism.

Suggested readings

1. Wikipedia, the free encyclopedia
2. Basic Laboratory Methods in Medical Parasitology by WHO 1991.
3. Training Manual on Diagnosis of Intestinal Parasites 2004.
4. Soulsby EJL (1982) Helminths, arthropods and protozoa of domesticated animals, 7th ed, Bailliere and Tindal, London, UK.

2

Present Status of Small Animal Farming and Role of Sheep Husbandry Department in Socio-economic Upliftment of Rural People

Nazam Khan[1] and Vikas Mahajan[2]

[1&2]Assistant Professor, *Division of ILFC*, Faculty of Veterinary Sciences & Animal Husbandry, SKUAST-Jammu-181102

Introduction

Mankind has been utilizing different animal species from the dawn of civilization for a variety of purposes *viz.*, production of milk, meat, wool, egg and leather. Apart from these, various animal species are also used for draught power, companionship, entertainment, research experimentation, sports, security etc. Livestock sector plays a crucial role in rural economy and livelihood. As per report of the working group on animal husbandry and dairying, 11th five year plan: 2007-12, the livestock sector employs eight percent of the countries labour force, including many small and marginal farmers, women and landless agricultural workers. Milk production alone involves more than 30 million small producers, each raising one or two cows or buffaloes. The organic fertilizer produced by the sector is an important input to crop production and dung from livestock is widely used as fuel in rural areas. Livestock also serves as an insurance substitute, especially for poor rural households; it can easily be sold during time of distress.

Indian livestock sector is one of the largest in the world with a holding of 11.6% of world livestock population. Contribution of livestock and fisheries sectors to the national economy in terms of Gross Domestic Product (GDP) is 4.1 and 0.8%, respectively. Agriculture and allied sector contributed about 15.1% to the total GDP. Out of the total agricultural GDP, livestock sector contributed about 27.25% during 2012-13. The livestock sector is an important source of foreign exchange too and is performing well in the manner of production, value addition and export of dairy, fishery, wool, poultry and other products.

The economy of Jammu and Kashmir (J&K) is still agriculture dependent and is the main occupation of majority of the rural people who earn their livelihood from it. Census figures 2011 signify that about 73% of the population lives in rural areas and are associated with agriculture and allied sectors including livestock rearing as main occupation.

J&K State is ideally suited for rearing of sheep and goats owing to its agro-climatic and geo-physical conditions. The pastoral area of state lie both in sub-tropical zone of Jammu, temperate, sub-alpines and alpine areas of both Jammu and Kashmir divisions. Nature which has bestowed this state with high mountains to low hills and vast meadows, provide enormous scope and excellent atmosphere for sheep and goat rearing. This sector is emerging as important growth leverage to state economy and its share to Gross State Domestic Products is also increasing. As per 19th Livestock census, 2012 (GOI, 2014), the total livestock population is 512.05 million. The share of total sheep and goat in the country is 65.06 million (12.71%), and 135.17 million (26.40%) numbers, respectively. However, J&K state stands in the 5th position with regard to Sheep population in the country. The percentage share of total sheep population-2012 of J&K is 3.39 million (5.21%). But, the percentage share of total goat population-2012 of J&K is 2.02 million (1.49%) and ranks 15th in India (Table 1).

In India, total wool production has increased from 27.5 million kg (1950-51) to 46.1 million kg (2012-13). Nearly 71% of the production of wool is contributed by Ram while Ewe and Lamb contributes 25% and 4%, respectively. Among states, wool production is maximum in Rajasthan followed by Karnataka, Jammu & Kashmir, Andhra Pradesh and Gujarat (BAHS, 2014). During the year 2011-12, the total wool production estimated for the State was 75.30 lakh kg which consisted of 61.59 lakh kg (81.79%) from cross-breed sheep and 13.71 lakh kg (18.20%) of local-breed Sheep (ISS, 2011-12). Also, the average wool yield per annum is 26.22 kg for cross-breed sheep and 17.50 kg for local-breed sheep. In other words, total availability of wool per person per annum is

629.98 gm for the state as a whole which included 515.28 gm from cross-breed sheep and 114.70 gm from local-breed sheep.

Likewise, total meat production in India is 5.9 million tonnes. Nearly 45% of the production of meat is contributed by poultry alone whereas contribution of goat and sheep to total meat production is 16% and 7%, respectively (BAHS, 2014). Andhra Pradesh produces maximum meat from sheep and poultry while West Bengal ranks first in goat meat production. The availability of meat in India is only about 15g/person/day against the ICMR recommendation of 30g/person/day. As per the Integrated Sample Survey Report (ISS), 2011-12, total estimated meat production of State was worked out to be 322.78 lakh kg consisting of 80.79% of Red Meat (260.76 lakh kg) and 19.21% of White Meat (62.02 lakh kg) and there is 4.47% growth of meat production. The meat availability was worked out to be 2.70 kg per person per year.

Table 1. Rank of sheep and goat population in India

Livestock	First rank country in world	India's rank in world	J&K rank in India
Sheep	China	2nd	5th
Goat	India	1st	15th

Source: BAHS (GOI). 2014

The importance of small ruminants can be established from the fact that it provides numerous food and non-food items to the people which are presented underneath:

i. **Food:** It provides food items *i.e.* milk and meat for human consumption.

ii. **Fibre and skins:** It also contributes to the production of wool, hair, hides, etc.

iii. **Draft:** Small ruminants are being extensively used to transport goods (small quantity) in hilly terrains as alternative to transport goods.

iv. **Dung and other animal waste materials:** Dung and other animal wastes serve as very good farm yard manure.

v. **Storage:** These are considered as "moving banks" because of their potentiality to dispose off during emergencies. They serve as capital and in cases of landless agricultural laborers, many times, it is the only capital resource they possess. It serves as an asset and in case of emergencies as guarantee for availing loans from the local sources such as money lenders in the villages.

vi. **Weed control:** Small ruminants are also used in biological control of bushes, plants and weeds.

vii. **Cultural:** They offer security to the owners and also add to their self esteem.

viii. **Sports / recreation:** People also use the rams for competition and sports.

ix. **Companion animals:** Small ruminants are known for their faithfulness and are being used as companions since time immemorial.

Role of small ruminants in farmers' economy

It plays an important role in the economy of farmers. The farmers in India maintain mixed farming system *i.e.,* a combination of crop and livestock where the output of one enterprise becomes the input of another enterprise thereby realize the resource efficiency. It serves the farmers in different ways.

1. **Income**: It is a source of subsidiary income for many families in India especially the resource poor who maintain few heads of animals. It serves as source of income during emergencies to meet exigencies like marriages, treatment of sick persons, children education, repair of houses etc. The animals also serve as moving banks and assets which provide economic security to the owners.
2. **Employment:** A large number of people in India being less literate and unskilled depend upon agriculture for their livelihoods. But agriculture being seasonal in nature could provide employment for a maximum of 180 days in a year. The land less and less land people depend upon livestock especially small ruminants for utilizing their labour during lean agricultural season.
3. **Food:** Its products such as milk, meat, etc. are an important source of animal protein to the members of the livestock owners.
4. **Social security:** These animals offer social security to the owners in terms of their status in the society. The families especially the landless which own animals are better placed than those who do not. Gifting

of animals during marriages is a very common phenomenon in different parts of the country. Rearing of animals is a part of the Indian culture. Animals are used for various socio-religious functions. Small ruminants are often sacrificed during festive seasons.

5. **Draft:** Small ruminants are being extensively used to transport goods (small quantity) in hilly terrains as alternative to transport goods.
6. **Dung:** Dung and other animal wastes serve as very good farm yard manure.

Role of sheep husbandry department in socio-economic upliftment of rural masses

The sheep husbandry has a major role in the development of small ruminant sector and upgrading of the socio-economic status of the rural masses in the state especially the average farmers. These departments are disseminating information by organizing the workshop, seminars, village level interaction with the different grades of socio-economic status of the people associated with the sector. These departments has been working with a mission to explore/adopt/introduce/promote/organize/undertake all activities viable for overall improvement of small ruminants for better productivity/output and subsequently create gainful self-employment avenues. The main aims and objectives of department are:

- To improve the production of wool, mutton, pashmina and chevon both qualitatively and quantitatively so as to improve the socio-economic status of sheep rearing communities on one hand and to meet the demand of wool and mutton to maximum level on other hand by way of extensive cross breeding programme.
- To study the problems of sheep husbandry sector in respect of feeding, management & disease control and to implement the programmes accordingly.

To increase the wool production, department has promoted cross breeding of local sheep with fine wool breeds like Merino in Kashmir and Rambouillet in Jammu division. As the major chunk of Sheep population of Jammu division is migratory in nature, this policy is being continued till date in these migratory, semi-migratory and stationary flocks of colder regions of the state. Due to introduction of superior fine wool germplasm in these areas about 65% sheep population has attained desired type of crossbred wool with subsequent increase in body weight.

Likewise to boost up mutton production, Dorper breed of sheep has been introduced in the state (plain border belts of Kathua, Rajouri, Jammu and Samba districts of the division). Department has also introduced an **Innovative Pilot Study Project on Embryo Transfer Technology** at Sheep Breeding Farm, Panthal to give boost to overall productivity of sheep sector in the state in which frozen embryos of Dorper and Rambouillet sheep are implanted in surrogate ewes.

For development of goat sector, to narrow down the gap between demand and supply of meat, the Department has introduced **Beetal breed.** To achieve the same, beetal bucks are being purchased from progressive breeders of Kathua district, Gurdaspur district of Punjab and also from Central Sheep Breeding Farm, Hisar (Haryana). These bucks are distributed among the breeders of Jammu, Samba, Kathua and Rajouri belt for improvement of their local goats so as to increase the milk and meat production. A dairy goat farm, Rajbagh is being maintained on pure beetal goats, breeding is maintained by department. Also, Kagani bucks are being purchased from progressive goat breeders of Rajouri, Udhampur, Reasi, Jammu and Samba districts and provided to the breeders having Kagani goats so as to conserve the breed on pure lines and to check the inbreeding.

Activities of Sheep Husbandry Department for benefitting rural masses

Germplasm Production Centres (Breeding Farms): The Sheep husbandry department Jammu has established six Sheep breeding farms and one dairy goat farm in Jammu division, which serve as Ram/Buck mother farms where quality germplasm is produced and distributed to private breeders through extension agencies of the department for up-gradation of their livestock.

Field Activities: The field activities of the department are controlled by the Joint Director, Extension, Sheep husbandry department Jammu. The field organizations are headed by the District sheep husbandry officers at district level, Block Veterinary Officers at block level. In addition, to cater to the need of migratory flocks, two ISD migratory

Projects are functioning in Jammu division and are controlled by the respective Assistant Project Officers. To meet the emergencies a mobile unit is functioning in the Joint Directorate of Extension.

The basic unit of extension work in the field is the Sheep Extension Centres (SECs). At present 484 SECs including 60 SECs opened with internal arrangement are catering to the needs of sheep and goat breeders. The staff of the centers is engaged in the overall development of sheep and goat sector in the area by extending breeding coverage, health care facilities, educating the sheep breeders about the scientific and improved rearing and management of sheep and providing all other necessary facilities. In case of the migratory center the staff of each center also moves along with the sheep and goat rearers and remains at alpines looking after the sheep and goats and return to plains with downward migration of livestock. These centers are scattered throughout the length and breadth of the province. Also detailed knowledge regarding basic scientific management practices *viz.*, rearing, feeding, vaccination, deworming, *etc.* of small ruminant farming are delivered by veterinary professionals to rural masses for their social upliftment.

Health Care: The sheep and goat flocks of breeders are being provided with various health care facilities *viz.*, deworming against internal parasitic infestation, dipping against ecto-parasites and treatment against various ailments. In addition vaccination is being performed against dreadful bacterial and viral diseases such as clostridial infections, FMD, Sheep Pox and PPR.

Disease Investigation Laboratory (DIL): The improvement of sheep with exotic germplasm has appreciably increased wool and mutton production, but the crossbred animals have become prone to diseases of economic importance. In order to have surveillance over various types of infections, the role of disease investigation laboratories and mini laboratories at District level has increased many folds. These laboratories are making all out efforts to check the disease outbreaks in field and farm livestock laying stress on prophylactic measures.

Fleece Testing Laboratory (FTL): In order to watch the improvement in wool quality and quantity, one FTL has been created, where wool samples from breeding stocks are collected and analyzed.

Sheep and Wool Workers Training: A training to newly selected stock assistants is provided by department. In addition, refresher training programmes are being launched for para-vets where they are being provided with latest technical knowledge and managemental practices.

Machine shearing / Training Programme: To have longer uniform staple length and higher wool yield, department has launched machine shearing programme for sheep flocks of breeders which has many advantages over conventional methods of hand shearing.

Publicity and Extension Activities: To have latest technical knowledge the sheep and goat rearers are being educated through various training programmes/awareness camps organized by the Department, besides distributing publicity/extension material in shape of pamphlets, brochures, posters, booklets, *etc.*, in Urdu/Hindi to the breeder community.

Fodder Resources: The feed and fodder has a significant bearing on the production of livestock. The agriculture activities of the department are supervised by the Deputy Director, feed & fodder. The agriculture wing of the department is engaged in cultivation of improved varieties of fodder at different farms and field organizations having the qualities of high volumes, biomass and digestible nutrients. The department has one Fodder Development Farm at Lam. The fodder produced at this farm is supplied to other farms to meet their requirement for feeding of the government livestock. This farm also caters to the need of sheep farms of Kashmir division.

Apart from above activities of sheep husbandry department, it also provides different employment generation schemes which are presented below:

A. State Sector Mini Sheep Farm Scheme (50 Ewes+ 2 Rams)

Particulars	Description
Sponsored by	State government
Description	Establishment of credit linked mini sheep farms of 50 Ewes and 2 Rams at cost of Rs. 2.38 lacs for unemployed youth of State. Margin Money of Rs. 0.38 lakh to be born by beneficiary. Rs. 2.00 lakhs credit through J&K bank Backend subsidy of Rs. 0.60 lakh to be paid by sheep husbandry department to concerned branch of J&K bank. Employment generation for two persons on establishment of unit.
Beneficiaries	Small marginal farmers, agriculture labourers, entrepreneurs and unemployed youth of State.
Benefit type	Rs. 0.60 lakh backend subsidy
Eligibility criteria	Possession of minimum wherewithal *viz.*, land, grazing rights, etc. Experience/ knowledge of trade Willingness to undergo mandatory training in management, record keeping etc. Willingness to invest margin money.
How to avail	Interested beneficiaries to apply to concerned District Sheep Husbandry Officers. Selection of beneficiaries by committee under Chairmanship of Additional District Development Commissioner.

3

Care and Management of Dairy Animals

Asma Khan and M. Rashid
Faculty of Veterinary Sciences & Animal Husbandry, SKUAST-Jammu-181102

Livestock sector has emerged as one of the key components of agricultural growth in developing countries in last few decades. This sector plays a significant role in the economic progress of India as it contributes 26% to the agricultural GDP and provides employment to around 18 million people. Over 70% of the rural households in India depends on livestock farming for supplementary income and is considered as an important instrument in poverty alleviation. It provides the major extra contribution to agriculture through manure, fuel fertilizer, apart from meat and milk that grant a regular supplementary income and employment not only to producers but also to huge size of the population engaged in secondary and tertiary business related to livestock. The economy of Jammu and Kashmir is also agriculture dependent and is the main occupation of majority of the rural people who earn their livelihood from it. Census figures 2011 signify that about 73% of the population of J&K lives in rural areas and are associated with agriculture and allied sectors including livestock rearing as main occupation. It is estimated that livestock and its derived foods and other products contribute about 6.13% to this Gross State Domestic Product (GSDP) in the year 2010-11.

India is endowed with the largest livestock population in the world (about 57.3% of the world's buffalo population and 14.7% of the cattle population). Whereas, estimated livestock population of the state is 155.87 lakhs in which large ruminants share is 24.95% (31.19 lakh cattle and 7.70 lakh buffalo). The total milk production in the country is 155 million tonnes during 2015-16; however the demand is expected to increase to 180 million tonnes by 2020. Also, estimated milk production for the State is 1609.25 thousand MTs and the demand of high milk production is true for state also. To achieve this demand annual growth rate in milk production has to be increased. Despite of this production, J&K is still importing huge bulk of animal products from the neighboring states viz. Rajasthan, Punjab, Haryana, etc. Thus, there is a tremendous scope/ potential for increasing the milk production through profitable dairy farming.

Also it provides employment throughout the year in comparison to agriculture which is mostly seasonal. Various technical and commercial aspects of dairy farming are dealt underneath in following subheadings:

- Breed selection
- Nutrition/Feeding management
- Housing management
- Reproduction management
- Health management
- General management (includes economics also)

Breed selection

Selection of Animals for Foundation Stock

Preferred breeds of cattle for dairy purpose are:

Exotic breeds: Holstein Friesian, Jersey, Brown Swiss.

Local breeds: Sahiwal, Red Sindhi, Tharparkar, Hariana, Gir, Ongole, Kankrej.

Crossbred cows: Karan Swiss, Karan Fries, Frieswal.

For buffaloes, preferred breeds are Murrah and Nilli ravi

The animals for constituting the foundation herd may be accessible from organized farms, private dairy farms and farmer herds. The following consideration should be kept in mind:

- Purchase dairy heifers or just calved cows with female calf in phases over a period of one year.
- Preference may be given to the breeds suitable to the agro-climatic region where dairy farm is established.

- Production records may be available on institutional herds, while very little information is available with farmers. Therefore, for purchasing milch animals, due weightage should be given to the quantity of milk produced in two consecutive milking depending upon the stage of lactation, breed type, age, pedigree and health status (disease free) of the animal.

While selection, the following points should be kept in mind

- Animal should have wide deep body, balanced standing on legs with thighs wide apart, loose and pliable skin, long tail and docile temperament;
- Body capacity- long straight back, wide barrel and deep heart girth;
- Mammary system- well attached large symmetrical udder, prominent milk well and tortuous milk veins, and small sized well-spaced teats.

Choose breeds and animals well suited to the local environment and farming system. It reduces the risks to productivity posed by animal health and welfare problems. Of particular relevance is the animal's ability to adapt to climatic extremes, feed quality, local parasites (especially ticks) and their acquired resistance to endemic disease. Animals introduced from different locations may be vulnerable to endemic diseases in the new location due to lack of previous exposure and the development of immunity.

Nutrition/Feeding management

Amount of nutrients required by animals are different for different phases of animal (viz. growth, lactation, work, pregnancy etc). The feeds available and production as well as physiological status of animal changes frequently. Therefore, it is necessary to compute ration for animals of different classes under different feeding conditions we have. The data comprising a feeding standard and feed composition are useful as a guideline in computation of ration and are presented in Tables 1,2,3,4,5.

Table 1. Nutrients required for growing cattle per head per day (Growth Requirement)

Live Wt (Kg)	Daily Wt Gain (g)	DCP (Kg)	TDN (Kg)
45	300	0.15	0.8
70	500	0.22	1.3
100	500	0.28	1.9
200	500	0.40	3.0
300	450	0.47	4.0
400	450	0.48	5.0

Table 2. Nutrients required for maintenance of adult cattle per head per day

Live Wt (kg)	DCP (kg)	TDN (kg)	Calcium (g)	Phosphorus (g)
350	0.227	2.70	8	8
400	0.254	3.03	9	9
450	0.282	3.37	10	10
500	0.296	3.69	11	11
550	0.336	3.71	12	12

Table 3. Nutrients required for milk production (per kg of milk) to be added to maintenance requirement (Production Allowance)

Fat % in milk	DCP (Kg)	TDN (Kg)	Calcium (g)	Phosphorus (g)
4.0	0.045	0.316	2	1.4
5.0	0.051	0.363	2	1.4
6.0	0.057	0.411	2	1.4
8.0	0.069	0.506	2	1.4
10.0	0.081	0.602	2	1.4

Table 4. Nutrients required for working cattle per head per day

Live Wt (Kg)	Normal work		Heavy work	
	DCP (Kg)	TDN (Kg)	DCP (Kg)	TDN (Kg)
400	0.45	4.0	0.57	4.8
500	0.56	4.9	0.71	6.4
600	0.66	5.8	0.84	7.2

Table 5. DCP & TDN content (Kg/100 Kg DM) of some common fodder & concentrates

Name of Fodder	DCP (Kg)	TDN (Kg)	Name of Concentrate	DCP (Kg)	TDN (Kg)
Green Fodders			**Grains and Seeds**		
Cereals: Jowar	2.4	56.6	Bajra	4.6	70.9
Maize	2.6	53.8	Guar	22.1	69.8
Oat	3.2	56.8	Pigeon pea	17.1	77.7
Hybrid Napier	5.8	52.5	Cotton seed	14.1	67.2
Legumes: Lucerne	19.3	69.7	**Oil seed Cakes**		
Berseem	14.2	63.9	Ground nut cake	37.8	82.0
Cabbage	9.3	52.9	Cotton seed cake	15.6	57.07
Cauliflower	9.0	73.5	**Cereal byproducts**		
Silage: Jowar	1.5	54.7	Maize bran	7.6	88.4
Hybrid Napier	3.3	48.7	Wheat bran	9.3	70.4
Dry Fodders			Rice bran	6.0	55.0
Jowar straw	1.5	59.3	Maize Gluten	40.5	71.3
Bajra straw	0.6	51.3	**Legume By-products**		
Wheat straw	0.2	56.8	Guar meal	35.1	73.9
			Sal seed cake	0.1	57.9
			Amul Dana	28-30	75.0

Pregnancy Allowance

During pregnancy, the animal should receive an extra allowance of 0.240 kg DCP and 1.4 kg TDN over and above maintenance and milk production. It is essential for the proper development of the fetus and in replacing the body stores of the energy that may have been utilized in the earlier part of lactation.

Feeding and watering requirement of Dairy Cattle

I. Feeding Roughage

On an average, dairy cattle consume dry roughage at the rate of 2.5% of their body weight. If the roughage is succulent, the consumption is 2 ½ to 3 times i.e. at the rate of 6 to 7.5 percent of body weight. If the cow weighs 400 kg, she will consume about 10 kg of dry roughage. If the roughage is succulent, she will take about 25 to 30 kg. The quantity of roughage consumption by an animal will vary from 1½ to 3½ % of its body weight according to the quality of the roughages. Good quality roughage is eaten more and *vice-versa.*

Dairy cattle should be fed good quality roughage as far as possible. Good quality roughage is low in fibre, leafier, greenish in color and is palatable. Dairy animals should be fed at least 33% of their total roughage requirement in form of succulent roughage. It contains factors of succulence i.e. certain unidentified nutritive factors, which lead to higher milk production. Preferably the ratio of leguminous to non-leguminous roughage should be 2:3.

II. Feeding Concentrates

The basal feed of dairy cattle is roughage. Moreover, the roughage is cheaper as compared to concentrates. Hence as far as possible, the nutrients required by dairy cattle should be given in the form of roughage. The concentrates should be fed to supply only their remaining nutrient requirement.

The quantity of concentrates to be fed daily to dairy animals will depend upon the quality and quantity of roughage fed to them. With good quality roughage, the concentrates to be fed will be less and *vice-versa*. So by feeding better quality roughages, we can curtail concentrate requirement.

III. Feeding Minerals

Dairy cattle need minerals like calcium, sodium, potassium and phosphorus in relatively larger amounts, and iron, copper, iodine and cobalt etc., in traces. Ordinarily, dairy cattle receive all minerals from their normal ration in sufficient quantities, except for sodium, calcium and phosphorus. But in areas where the soil on which the forage crops are grown is deficient in any one or more of the above minerals, there may be deficiency of the same in the ration of animals. This deficiency should be corrected by feeding suitable mineral supplements.

Under ordinary condition, the dairy cattle are fed common salt mixed with the concentrates. If the roughage fed is non-leguminous, they may also be fed steam sterilized bone meal or any other calcium supplement. When leguminous roughage is fed to dairy cattle, supplying additional calcium through such supplement is not necessary. Now-a-days, several mineral mixtures are available in the market. They are mixed with concentrates. Extra mineral mixture is given to high producing cows.

IV. Providing Water

Water constitutes over 70% of the animal body and over 85% of the milk. It is therefore not surprising that the daily consumption of water is greater than that of the any other nutrient. Lack of water will retard growth and reduce production.

As a general rule, allow 5 parts of water for each part of air dry feed. Equal amount of water is also needed for washing of animals, utensils and sheds.

Under average conditions the (a) Beef cattle, Dry cows, Bullocks etc. may drink 5 to 8 litres of water/100 kg body wt. and (b) Lactating Dairy cows may drink 5 to 8 litres/100 kg body wt for maintenance plus 3 litres of water per kg of milk produced.

V. Calculation of Feed and Water Requirement for a Dairy Herd

From the herd register or roll call register, collect the information of different classes of animals in the herd. From this information calculate the equivalent adult units in the herd. The adult units give rough idea about feed and water requirement, wherein different classes of animals are compared with an adult cow of average body weight. Under average condition, following guideline is used for calculation of adult units.

1 Cow	=	1 Adult Unit (AU)
1 Bull	=	1.25 AU
1 Bullock	=	1 AU
4 Calves	=	1 AU
3 Indian heifers from 1 to 2 yrs of age	=	1 AU
2 Indian heifers from 2 to 3 yrs age	=	1 AU
2 Crossbred heifers above 1 year of age	=	1 AU

Now, from the total adult units calculate the feed and water required in the herd daily,

Housing Management

1. Conventional Housing or Stanchion Barn

In this system, the animals are tied throughout the day and night in a completely enclosed structure or barn. Feeding, watering, milking, treatment etc is carried out at the same place. This system is followed in countries having cold climate such as European countries. Facilities for heating or cooling the internal air are also provided in the barn through heaters or coolers and used according to the season. Management is also mostly through automation.

2. Loose Housing System

Here the animals are kept loose all the while, except a temporary tying at the time of milking and treatment. Facilities of suitable manger under the shed and water-trough in paddock under the tree-shade are provided to the animals for free access to feed, water and rest. This system is widely practiced in hot tropical countries including India due to its many advantages over conventional system. There are certain advantages viz. animals can move freely and are most comfortable to get feed, water, sunlight, exercise etc at their will, construction cost is less, expansion of buildings/sheds is easy, if required in future, sheds have flexible utility, labour saving - less labourers required for feeding, watering, cleaning etc. Also detection of heat, sickness and such problems is easy since the animals can manifest them through their behavior. But there are certain limitations also i.e. separate milking parlor is required, more labour is required for catching and handling of animals. Chances of spread of contagious disease are more and it is difficult to disinfect these sheds regularly and completely.

The floor space, feeding and watering space requirement for different categories of animals are presented in Table 6 and 7

Table 6. Floor Space requirement per animal as per BIS (Bureau of Indian Standard)

S. No.	Category of animals	Floor space required (sq.m.)		Maximum No. of animals/shed
		Under shed	*In paddock*	
1.	Cows	3.5	7.0	50
2.	Buffaloes	4.0	8.0	50
3.	Down calvers (Advanced pregnant cows/heifers)	12.0	12.0	Individual
4.	Breeding Bulls	1.0	2.0	30
5.	Young calves/Older calves	2.0	4.0	30

Table 7. Feeding and Watering Space requirements

S. No.	Category of animals	Feeding space/ animal (cm)	Watering space/ animal (cm)	Width of manger/ water-trough (cm)	Depth of manger/ water-trough (cm)
1.	Adult C/B	60-75	6.0-7.5	60	40
2.	Calves	40-50	4.0-4.5	40	15

Reproduction management

The various reproductive disorders that a dairyman may observe in his cows, their diagnosis and treatment is presented in Table 8. In India fertility in case of she-buffaloes during summer is generally assumed to be poor. This problem can be rectified by the use of vasectomised bull for heat detection. Moreover supplementation of minerals and antioxidants during summer has also positive effects on the conception rate. Pregnant cows and buffaloes should be transferred to individual calving pens at least 3-4 weeks before the expected date of calving. Veterinary aids should be preferred to handling by inexperienced quacks of all calving difficulties. However after calving, sanitation is the most important factor in overcoming breeding trouble.

Table 8. History, findings, diagnosis and treatment of infertility conditions in cows and she-buffaloes

Dairyman's history	Per rectal findings	Diagnosis	Treatment
Irregular heats			
Chronic buller or nymphomania	Follicular cysts on ovary		Rupture of cysts per rectum; parentrally
Shorter cycles (<21 days)	Ovaries normal-Presence of small corpus luteum (CL)	Progestrone insufficiency	200 mg progesterone on 1st to 5th day of cycle
Longer cycles (24-29 days or longer)	Active CL, but no pathology nor pregnant	Missed heat	Check for next heat by improving heat diagnosis
	Firmly organized CL	Failure of recession of CL	Parentral administration of estrogens
	Tract normal, CL small	Infantalism (in heifers)	Administration of estrogens and follicular stimulating hormone (FSH)
Regular heats, but animals fails to conceive	No pathology on palpation	Subclinical uterine infection	Pre or post-service antibiotic douche
		Delayed ovulation	Small dose of LH or progesterone
		Failure of fertilization	Above treatment
	Adhesions of ovarian bursa to ovaries-unilateral or bilateral	Bursal a dhesions	Try to break the adhesion, if breaking is impossible cull the animal, if CL is small use 200mg progesterone at the time of heat

	Spongy and enlarged oviduct or fallopian tubes adhesions too	Salphingitis accompanied by other pathology	Parentral and I/U antibiotic medication
Anoestrous (no heat)	Uterine horn gravid with foetus	Pregnancy	No interference
	Thick spongy uterine horn, pits on pressure, exudates from posterior of cervix, CL present	Metritis	Enucleate CL, estrogen administration and Lugol's iodine or antibiotic uterine douches
	No functional CL, small inactive ovaries, tract normal	Non-functional ovaries due to deficiency	Nutrition-check the deficiency by feeding balanced rations and cull old animals

Health management

The common diseases encountered in the farm are infectious diseases, parasitic diseases, deficiency diseases, metabolic diseases and injuries done to body by cuts, blows, falls, etc. These diseases can be prevented by adopting different measures such as isolation of sick animals, quarantine, vaccination, balanced feeding and accurate diagnosis. As soon as as an outbreak occurs, following points should be kept in mind:

- Segregate sick animals
- Adopt biosecurity measures i.e. stop all animals, animal products, vehicles and persons coming into and out of the farm.
- Avoid grazing in a common place.
- Ban all visitors to the farm.
- Provide foot dips containing disinfectants at the entry of farm and gear up sanitation and hygiene.

Vaccinate all animals as recommended or required by local animal health authorities

Vaccination is a useful tool to limit the impact of disease by increasing the immunity of the animal population to specific pathogens. Animal health authorities can provide dairy farmers with information about the specific vaccines which are recommended for their area. In some dairying regions, dairy farmers are required by law to vaccinate their stock against serious contagious diseases. The routinely used vaccination schedule is presented in Table 9

Table 9. Vaccination schedule of large ruminants

FMD						
Raksha	Indian Immunologicals	Inactivated tissue culture FMD virus strains O, A and Asia-1 adsorbed on Al $(OH)_3$gel and saponin as an adjuvant	3 ml in the mid-neck region, s/c (Vial: 30 ml)	4 months	2-4 weeks after primary vaccination	Every 6 months after booster and every 4 months in endemic areas
Raksha Ovac	-do-	Inactivated tissue culture FMD virus strains O, A, and Asia-1 adjuvanted with mineral oil	2 ml in the mid-neck region, deep i/m	4 months	9 months after primary vaccination	Annually
Haemorrhagic Septicemia (Galghotu/Ghurrka)						
Raksha HS	Indian Immunologicals	Formaldehyde inactivated culture of*Pasteurella multocida*adsorbed on aluminium hydroxide gel	2 ml, mid-neck region, s/c (Vial:100 ml)	6 months and above	Annually and in adverse climatic conditions like unseasonal rains and cyclones, *etc.*	Raksha HS

Compound Vaccines of FMD/HS/BQ						
Raksha biovac (FMD+HS)	Indian Immunologicals	FMD inactivated antigens against O, A, and Asia-1 strains and formaldehyde inactivated *Pasteurella multocida* culture mixed together in light mineral oil emulsion	3 ml, midneck, deep i/m (Vial: 30 ml)	4 months	9 months	Annually
Raksha triovac (FMD+HS+BQ)	-do-	FMD inactivated antigens against O, A, Asia-1 and formaldehyde inactivated *Pasteurella multocida* culture, inactivated *Clostridium chauvoei* culture mixed together in light mineral oil emulsion	3 ml, mid-neck, deep i/m (Vial: 30 ml)	4 months	9 months	Annually

Brucellosis						
Bruvax	Indian Immunologicals	Live *Brucella abortus*strain 19 freeze dried bacteria, each dose e" $40x10^9$ organisms	2 ml., s/c (Vial: 5 dose freeze dried vaccine with 10 ml sterile diluent)	4-8 months old serologically negative female calves	Bruvax	
Note: Only serologically negative female calves should be vaccinated with live B. abortus strain 19 while bulls and pregnant animals should not be vaccinated						
Depending upon prevalence in a given area, vaccination against following diseases may also be taken up Anthrax						
Raksha-Anthrax (Prophylactic only)	Indian Immunologicals	Suspension of live spores of attenuated non-capsulated strain of*B. anthracis* in 50% glycerinated saline, each dose e " $1x10^8$ viable spores	1 ml, i/m or s/c (Vial: 50 ml)	one month before grazing season or prior to the time the disease usually occurs	Raksha-Anthrax (Prophylactic only)	Indian Immunologicals
Note: Protect animals from overexertion 3 days following vaccination. Do not vaccinate the animal 60 days before slaughter						

Deworming

In hot and humid areas, it is almost essential to deworm livestock regularly. In adult animals deworming is done on examination of dung. All the animals should preferably be fasted for 24 hours before giving the anthelmintic. Young animals should preferably be dewormed every month with a suitable anthelmintic whereas older stock can be dewormed at 4-6 months interval. Some common and proven anthelmintics used are given in Table 10

Table 10. Common chemical anthelmintics used for control of internal parasites

Anthelmintic	Dose	Mode of administration	Remarks
Piperazine salt	0.2-0.4 g/kg body weight	Mixed in concentrate mixture or drinking water or oral dosing of individual animals followed by mild laxative if heavy infestation is expected	Most effective against ascarids and nodular worms
Thiabendazole	0.05-0.1 g/kg body weight	Mixed in feed or water or as an electuary or tablet	Effective against strongyles and other worms
Phenothiazine	70-90 g	Mixed in feed or water or as oral doses or tablets	Effective against strongylosis
Hexachlorethane	0.2-0.25 g/kg body weight	Preferably as a suspension with bentomite (4:1)	Effective against flukes and stomach worms

General management

Management of heifer

Better Care and Management of heifer will give high quality replacement stock to the dairy farm. Some recommendations are presented below:

- Feed the heifer sufficiently to produce normal growth. During the early stage, provide more protein than energy. Most heifers grow well if sufficient hay is provided.
- The heifers should be provided with a dry shelter free from drafts.
- Weight attained by heifers is more important than age for breeding time. Never bred a under sized heifer to avoid calving problems. Usually the heifer is bred to freshen at 24-30 months of age.
- Place the heifer in a separate shed about 6-8 weeks before she is due to calve.
- Feed 2 - 3 kg of concentrate daily and all the forage she eats.
- Before calving let the heifer becomes accustomed to handling and to the procedures used in the milking herd. Always handle her gently and with kindness.
- Maintenance of health among heifers is very important for proper growth.

Management of milch animal

- Provide green succulent forage together with leguminous hay or straw to the extent of animal can consume, so that all its maintenance requirements are met through forage only.
- Extra concentrate at the rate of 1 kg for every 2 to 2.5 liters of milk should be provided. Salt and mineral supplements should be given to maintain the lactation. Animals should be fed at regular intervals. *Ad lib* water should be provided thrice daily.
- Never frighten or excite the animals. Always treat them gently and with kindness.
- With proper feeding and care, a cow will come to heat within 16 days of calving. Do not with hold service unnecessarily after the signs of heat are noticed in a cow.
- By maintaining proper records of breeding and calving, a regular production of milk can be ensured.
- Regularity in milking is essential by full hand milking technique. Increase of milk in the udder will reduce further secretion of milk.
- Cows should be trained to let down milk without calf suckling. This will held to wean the calves early.

- Grooming of the cows and washing of the buffaloes before milking help in clean milk production.
- Wallowing of buffaloes or water spraying on their bodies will keep the buffaloes comfortable especially in summer.
- Common ailments should be properly detected and treated.
- Provide at least 60-90 days dry period between calvings. If the dry period is not sufficient, the milk yield is subsequent lactation will be reduced.
- Check for mastitis regularly.

4

Care and Management of Sheep and Goat

Nazam Khan and R.K. Sharma*
Assistant Professor, Division of ILFC, Faculty of Veterinary Sciences & Animal Husbandry, SKUAST-Jammu-181102
*Divison of Veterinary Nutrition

Small ruminant sector, after agriculture, is the second largest means for economic sustainability and livelihood in India. It contributed Rs. 32000 crore to the gross domestic product of India in 2012 -13 despite having a potential to contribute over Rs. 150,000 crore but there are certain lacunae in system which act as its growth inhibitor. Small ruminants are the main source for rural economies due to participation of women (70% of total) and weaker sections of the rural society. Thus there is urgent need for formulating policies to support the development of the small ruminant sector.

Sheep and goat husbandry is a tool for poverty alleviation of the rural masses because of wide adaptability with low investments, high fertility and fecundity, low feed and management costs, higher feed conversion efficiency, quick pay off and low risk in comparison to large ruminants. The above traits of small ruminants need to be exploited for economic upliftment of small farmers.

Also due to lack of supportive policies, the sector remains ignored and the farmers are deprived of the attainable economic benefits. The ICAR Institutions like Central Sheep and Wool Research Institute and Central Institute of Goat Research have been putting on good efforts to trigger a positive change in spite of low budgetary provisions, but lack of an organized technology transfer infrastructure restricts sustainable development in this sector. Thus there is a tremendous scope/potential for increasing the small ruminant production through profitable farming. Various technical aspects regarding above are presented underneath in detail.

Sheep

Sheep in India are mostly maintained on natural vegetation on common grazing lands, wastelands and uncultivated (fallow) lands, stubbles of cultivated crops and top feeds (tree loppings). Rarely are they kept on grain, cultivated fodder or crop residue. Sheep are mostly reared for wool and meat. Sheep skins and manure constitute important sources of earning, the latter particularly in southern India. Milk from sheep is of limited importance and that too in very limited areas of Jammu and Kashmir, Rajasthan and Gujarat. Indian sheep are not regarded as dairy sheep.

Unique characteristics of sheep

1. Strong herd instincts of sheep make them excellent ranch animals as they remain together in tight and easily managed flocks and do not disperse widely all over the available land, which would make it difficult to protect them from predators and difficult to round up.
2. Excellent ability to survive over a prolonged period of drought and semi-starvation.
3. Sheep have the ability to produce prime carcasses on roughage alone, thus they are well adapted to many areas unable to produce grain profitably.
4. The structure of their lips helps them to clean grains lost at harvest time, and thus convert waste feed into profitable products.
5. Less prone to extreme weather conditions, ectoparasites as well as other diseases.
6. Unique ever-growing fibre which allows ventilation and also protects the skin from the hot sun, rain and abrasions.
7. Sheep can also constrict or relax blood vessels in the face, legs and ear for control of heat loss.

Classification of indigenous breeds based on utility

Apparel wool breeds	Superior carpet Wool breeds	Coarse carpet Wool breeds	Hairy Meat breeds
Hissardale	Chokla	Malpura	Nellore
Niligiri	Nali	Sonadi	Hassan
Kashmir merino	Marwari	Muzzafarnagri	Mecheri
Avivastra	Magra	Jalauni	Kilakarsal
Bharat Merino	Jaisalmeri	Deccani	Madras Red
Hissardale	Pugal	Bellary	Trichy Black
	Pattanwadi	Coimbatore	Kenguri
	Tibetan	Chottanagpuri	Mandya
	Bonpala	Balangir	Vembur
	Gaddi	Ganjam	
	Rampur Bushari	Bhakarwal	
	Poonchi	Shahabadi	
	Karnah		

Exotic breeds

Fine wool breeds	Mutton breeds	Dual purpose	Pelt breeds
Merino	Suffolk	Corriedale	Karakul
Rambouillet	Southdown		
Polworth	Dorset		

Feeding of sheep

The feeding and grazing conditions vary from place to place. The most favorable grazing time is soon after the onset of monsoon till the onset of winter. Grazing resources become extremely poor during summer months. During this period supplementary feeding should be done. Sheep generally thrive well on pasture. Attention should be paid on pasture improvement and management. Rotational grazing should be followed to avoid worm infection and unthriftiness, and to ensure availability of good pasture all the time. The fodder should be conserved in the form of hay and silage for the lean period. Fodder trees should be planted in the pasture to provide shade and fodder during the lean period to the grazing flocks. Supplementary feeding of concentrate should be done depending upon the physiological status and availability of grazing resource in the pasture.

Water

Water requirement of sheep vary depending upon its physiological status and ambient temperature in different seasons. The sheep should be watered at least once a day at the rate of 2-3 litres per head per day. The requirement of water for crossbreds during summer months will be slightly more and may range between 5-6 litres. The younger ones may require 1-2 litres of water every day. Sheep breeds in arid regions have good adaptation to water restriction up to 48 hrs. Watering should be done in metallic troughs or cements channels. The flock should be weighed at least once in a week to the extent of at least 10% prior to being turned out for grazing. This work may be distributed over the week.

1. **Feeding lambs up to two weeks**: There is no feed equal to the ewe's milk for putting rapid gains on young lamb because dam's milk yield is closely related to early growth of lamb. Lambs depend entirely on dam's milk up to 2 weeks. Colostrum is rich in fat, protein, vitamins etc. and contains antibodies to protect the lamb from infections. If the ewes are fed good ration during the last six weeks of gestation, it enhances milk production.

Feeding lambs beyond two weeks : The recommended rations are given below:

Feed ingredients (%)	Pre-weaning period (upto 3 months)	(3-6 months)	Finisher
Ground maize	65	27	25
Groundnut cake	10	35	20
Wheat bran	12	35	52
Fish meal	10	-	-
Common salt	1	1	1
Min. mix.	2	2	2
Expected growth rate per day (gms)	110-125	100-120	100-120

Rate of feeding/day (approx)

	Body weight	Concentrate (gms)		Roughage
		Legume is available	Legume not available	
1	12-15	50	300	ad lib
2	15-25	100	400	ad lib
3	25-35	150	600	ad lib

2. **Feeding suckling ewes:** During suckling period, ewes should be fed good milk producing ration. She should be fed good legume hay or oat hay with little or no grain for a week. After she's milking freely and her bowels are functioning normally with no sign of constipation, the amount of grains may be increased. If pasture is available, hay is not needed. The following rations can be used :-

	Feed ingredients	Ration-I	Ration-II
1	Grain mixture	400gm	400gm
2	Legumes hay	700gm	1400gm
3	Green fodder/silage	1400gm	-

3. **Feeding adult sheep :** Roughage part may be taken care by grazing, but 150 gm of concentrate (as for suckling ewes) with mineral mixture and salt must be fed.

   Energy: Adult – Non pregnant sheep – 93 K cal. ME/kg $w^{0.75}$

   Lactating - 102 K cal. ME / kg. $w^{0.75}$

Protein – DCP requirement – 1g for every 1 kg $w^{0.75}$ live weight (adult non pregnant) Increases by 50% during pregnancy and 100% during lactation.

Flushing

Ewes which are to be bred should be underfed for about 45 days prior to breeding in order to prevent fat accumulation which reduces fertility. Two weeks prior to breeding, the ewes should be fed about 150-200 gm concentrate mixture daily along with good quality forages (cowpea, oat, doob grass, berseem). It conditions the animal and induces maturation of more number of follicles, and thus improves conception and twinning rate.

4. **Feeding breeding rams:** Good quality green fodders like maize, cowpea, oat, doob grass, lucerne, berseem etc. would meet all requirements of breeding rams. If forages fed are of poor quality like straw or sorghum hay, then 150-200 gms concentrate should be fed daily.

Area-specific mineral mixture: Area specific mineral mixtures (ASMM) for sheep and goats of semi-arid region of Rajasthan have been developed for improving health, reproduction and production level. The ASMM is available in both pelleted and powder form. The later is having advantage of delivering the micronutrients in more complete and in quantifiable manner.

5. **Complete feed block (CFB):** The complete feed block of roughage and concentrate mixture was prepared in 70:30 ratios with 5% of molasses for easy binding. The blocks have many advantages like ease in transport, palatable in nature, lower in space requirement for storage and reduced losses during transport. Use of feed block to sheep reduces the cost per kg gain by 38% as compared to the control diet (grass hay and concentrate). CFB reduces the bulk density by 33% and can be stored up to 2 yrs in dry weather without deterioration in nutrients.

Vaccination in sheep

Disease	Age and booster doses	Route	Remarks
FMD	6-8 weeks;repeat every 6-9 months	s/c or i/m depending on the vaccine	-
H.S	3-4 months;repeat annually	1 ml s/c	May/ June
Sheep pox	3 months	s/c	-
Tetanus	Tetanus toxoid	0.5 - 1 ml s/c or i/m	-
Anthrax	4-6 months; repeat annually	0.5 ml s/c at tail fold	In endemic areas
Enterotoxaemia	3-4 months, repeat after 15 days and then annually.	2.5 ml s/c	First two doses before august

Grazing management of sheep

Purpose: As pasture is a valuable fodder for sheep and the cheapest source of nutrients necessary for maintenance and production, proper grazing management and care of pastures is essential for ensuring higher yields.

Characteristics of sheep feeding under range conditions

Sheep have a small muzzle and split upper-lip which enables them to nibble tiny blades of vegetation which cannot be eaten by larger animals. Sheeps prefer small, tender grasses and chew food more thoroughly than cattle. The capacity of the sheep stomach is 15-16 litres and excess feeding can cause indigestion and they do not relish ripe grass. Sheep on pastures may consume 10-15 % more dry matter compared to stall feeding and daily grazing for 10-12 hours should be permitted to meet the dry matter requirements. Sheep usually relish leguminous fodder such as lucerne, cowpea, berseem etc. and rotation of pastures should be should be adopted to prevent under- or over-grazing. Growing lambs should be allowed to graze first, followed by pregnant and lactating ewes, and dry stock at the last (If cattle, sheep and goats are to graze on the same pasture, it will be desirable to allow goats first, followed by cattle and sheep, in that order). Even a good pasture does not meet the dietary requirements of advanced pregnant and lactating ewes, and hence additional concentrate feed of 250-300 gm/day should be given.

Pasture improvement and management

Pasture lands in India are poor and meager and need to be improved by protecting them from biotic factors, conserving good natural grasses, choosing the best fodder trees and shrubs, removing nonedible grasses, weeds and shrubs, and re-seeding with nutritious and perennial grasses and legumes. Natural legumes like *Rhynochosia minima, Indigofera endecaphylla* and *Tribulus terrestris* are very useful and should be preserved. Grazing lands should be re-seeded with nutritious perennial grasses like *Cenchrus ciliaris, Cenchrus setigerus, Lasiruss indicus* and *Dichanthium annulatum* in arid and semiarid plains; Sehimanervosum in sub-humid plains; and fescue, rye grass and kikyu grass in the temperate and sub-temperate regions. Perennial legumes like *Dolichos lablab, Clitoriaternatea, Macropteliumatropurpureum, Atylosiascara-bacoides* and *Stylosanthus* species should be incorporated in the regenerated or reseeded pastures. Combined production of grass and legumes can increase forage production by 20-30 per cent as compared to that of grass alone. The legumes, besides being rich in protein content, are more palatable and digestible, enrich the soil by nitrogen fixation, and help in checking soil erosion. During the first year of pasture establishment, grazing should not be allowed; the fodder must be harvested, conserved as hay, and fed during the lean period. Rotational grazing, i.e. dividing the pasture into four equal compartments and allowing grazing sequentially, helps the grasses to regenerate, checks soil erosion caused by over-grazing and allows agricultural operations to be carried out. Pastures should be top dressed with sufficient quantities of farmyard and inorganic fertilizers at regular intervals. Protection of pasture, removal of undesirable bushes and weeds, soil and water conservation, application of fertilizers, proper stocking rate and grazing system (rotational or deferred rotational) are essential components of good pasture management.

Silviculture

1. Fodder trees serve as a potential source of feed for sheep during December to June when the grazing resources become scarce.
2. Fodder trees also provide shade during summer, check soil erosion and improve soil texture.
3. Fodder trees should be planted in well-managed pastures after the first monsoon rains at a spacing of 20 x 10 metres (approx. 50 trees/hectare).
4. Lopping can be done twice a year in Oct-Nov (conserved) and May-Jun (fed green) in such a manner that the top branches are left in situ; yielding about 8-10 quintals of good quality green fodder.
5. The pods of many trees, especially babool (*Acacia arabica*) and khejri (*Prosopis cineraria*) are very nutritious and palatable, and serve as a good source of feed for flushing ewes.

Reproductive management in sheep

Reproductive management, comprising of detection of estrus, mating, identifying pregnant animals, care of pregnant animals, care at parturition and care of the male, plays a major role in the profitability of a sheep or goat farm. Effective managerial interventions can increase reproductive health, incidence of twinning/triplets and lamb/kid livability.

Age at mating: Sheep normally attain good growth at about 24 months (range 18-36) of age. Breeding too young ewes results in more weaklings and higher lamb losses. It is desirable to use rams for mating from the age of 2 years till the age of 7 years.

Mating season and estrus cycle: Sheep are seasonally polyestrus. In India, there are three main breeding seasons viz. summer (Mar-Apr), autumn (Jun-Jul) and post-monsoon (Sep-Oct). In general, higher fertility is observed in autumn season in the plains and in summer season in the hilly areas. The ewes usually come in heat about 2 months after lambing. The duration of the estrus cycle is 17 days (range 14-19) and heat period lasts for 27 hours (2-60). Ovulation occurs about 12 hours before the end of heat period.

Preparations for breeding

1. *Flushing*: Feeding extra grain or lush pasture 2-3 weeks prior to the breeding season for the purpose of increasing the number of ova shed from the ovary and increase the incidence of twinning. Feeding about 250 gms grains daily to each ewe results in an increase in the lamb crop by about 10-20 per cent.
2. *Tagging*: This refers to the shearing the locks of wool and dirt from the dock of the ewes, thus facilitating mating by the ram.
3. *Eyeing*: This refers to the clipping of excess wool around the eyes to prevent wool blindness in some breeds.
4. *Ringing*: This refers to shearing of wool from the body of the ram, especially in the neck, belly and sheath region prior to the breeding season.

Detection of estrus: As sheep in heat show few external indications of estrus other than standing to be mounted, heat is generally detected with the help of a teaser. Wet paint (dye mixed in grease or linseed oil) can be smeared on the brisket of the teaser ram to spot the ewes in estrus. The colour of the dye should be changed every 16-18 days so that the repeaters can be discovered. Other indications of estrus are vulvar swelling, frequent urination, restlessness and reduced appetite.

Mating: As far as possible, rams should be kept away from the ewes and the two should be brought together only for breeding. Natural breeding is done either by flock mating, pen mating or hand mating.

- In flock mating, breeding rams are usually turned out in the flock during the mating season at the rate of 2-3 per cent of the ewes all through day and night.
- In semi-flock breeding or pen mating, rams are turned out for service with the flock in the pen during night, and confined and stall-fed or grazed separately during the day time in order to conserve their energy and give them rest.
- Hand mating is practiced when exotic purebred sires are used, or when it is considered desirable to extend the services of the ram over much larger flocks.

Identifying pregnant ewes: Identification of pregnant ewes is essential for the re-breeding of empty ewes and efficient management of pregnant ewes. Pregnancy can be diagnosed by observing for cessation of estrus cycle, abdominal ballotment (from third month onwards) and by means of a chemical test.

Procedure: Mix 5 ml of urine sample and 5 ml of 1% Barium chloride solution. Turbidity indicates pregnancy whereas clear solution indicates non-pregnant condition.

Feeding of goats

Goats generally produce more milk than a cow from the same quantity of nutrients. The nutrient conversion efficiency for the production of milk in goats is 45.71 per cent, whereas a dairy cow averages 38 per cent. It has been observed that goats are 4.04 per cent superior to sheep, 7.90 per cent superior to buffaloes, and 8.60 per cent superior to cows in crude fibre utilization. The goat uses more useless feeds for its maintenance than a cow.

The secret of successful feeding is in devising a cheap and efficient ration. While preparing a ration for goats, factors like bulk, palatability, availability, price and digestibility should be considered along with the nutritive quality of the feed. Abundant clean, fresh water, changed every morning and evening should be made available to goats at all times. Some of the most serious diseases of goats result from the drinking of dirty water from shallow pools. Water troughs should be thoroughly washed at least twice a month. Goats in milk require more water than dry goats and should be watered regularly at least three times a day.

Feeding habits: Goats are sensitive animals with peculiar feeding habits. By the means of their mobile upper lips and very prehensile tongue, goats are able to graze on very short grass and to browse on foliage not normally eaten by other domestic livestock. Unlike sheep, goats relish eating aromatic plants in areas of scarce food supply and hence can penetrate deep into deserts. They are fastidious about cleanliness and like frequent change in the feed. Feeds given must be clean and fresh, since goats eat nothing that is dirty or foul-smelling. They dislike wet, stale or trampled fodder. For this reason, it is advisable to feed them in hay-racks or hang the feed in bundles from a peg in the wall or from a branch of a tree. Double-sided portable hay-racks are the most suitable and convenient for stall feeding. It is preferable to serve them small quantities at a time; when served in large quantities at a time, they waste a lot of it by trampling.

Goats are very fond of leguminous fodders. They do not relish fodder like sorghum/maize silage or straw. Goats do not relish hay prepared from forest grasses, even if cut in early stages, but very much relish hay prepared from leguminous crops. Some of the common green roughages liked by goats are : lucerne, berseem, napier grass, green arhar, cowpea, soyabean, cabbage and cauliflower leaves, shaftal, senji, methi, shrubs and weeds of different kinds; and leaves of trees such as babul, neem, ber, tamarind and pipal. The common dry fodders liked by goats are straws of arhar, urid, mung, gram, dry leaves of trees, and lucerne/berseem hays (which are the main forage crops for milch goats).

Nutrients required: The nutrients needed may be divided into maintenance, production and pregnancy requirements:-

a) **Maintenance ration**: As goats have a higher BMR than cattle, their maintenance requirements are higher. The maintenance requirement is 0.09 per cent DCP and 0.09 per cent TDN. For its size, a goat can consume substantially more feed than cattle or sheep, viz. 6.5-11 per cent of its body weight in dry matter when compared with 2.5-3 per cent for cattle or sheep. This means that the goat can satisfy its maintenance requirement and produce milk from forage alone.

b) **Production ration**: Requirements for the production of 1 litre of milk with 3 % and 4.5 % fat is 43 gm of DCP and 200 gm of starch equivalent (SE), and 60 gm of DCP and 285 gm of SE, respectively. The nutritional requirement of a goat weighing 50 kg and yielding 2 litres of milk with 4% fat may be met by feeding 400gm of concentrate mixture and 5 kg of berseem or lucerne. The ration should have 12-15 % protein content.

   The following concentrate mixtures may be used to feed the goat : (i) 1 part of wheat bran, 2 parts of maize grain, and 1 part of linseed cake, or (ii) 2 parts of maize grain, 1 part of barley, 2 parts of mustard-cake, and 2 parts of gram husk, or (iii) 1 part of wheat bran, 2 parts of barley grain, and 1 part of groundnut cake, or (iv) 2 parts of gram grain and 1 part of wheat bran. The above mixtures should also contain 2 % each of mineral mixture and salt.

c) **Pregnancy ration**: The foetal growth in the last 2 months of pregnancy is rapid and the metabolic rate of the goat rises rapidly. During this period, the content of ration should be increased to the level of production ration. A week before she kids, the doe should be provided with more succulent type of feed. For three or four days after kidding, the level of diet should be lowered and made more fibrous. This is necessary to minimize the shock to the goat's udder. After this period, the feeding should be done at a normal rate.

Feeding of kids: Immediately after birth, feed the young ones with colostrum and up to 3 days of birth keep dam with young ones for 2-3 days for frequent access of milk. After 3 days and up to weaning feed the kids with milk at 2 to 3 times a day. At about 2 weeks of age the young ones should be trained to eat green roughages and at one month of age the young ones should be provided with the concentrate mixture (Creep feed).

Composition of ideal creep feed

- Maize - 40%
- Ground nut cake - 30%

- Wheat bran - 10%
- Deoiled rice bran- 13%
- Molasses - 5%
- Mineral mixture- 2%
- Salt - 1% fortified with vitamins A, B2 and D3 and antibiotic feed supplements.

Feeding schedule for a kid/lamb from birth to 90 days

Age of kids/lambs	Dam's milk (ml)	Creep feed (grams)	Forage, green/day (gm)
1-3 days	Colostrum-300 ml, 3 feedings	-	-
4-14 days	350 ml, 3 feedings	-	-
15-30 days	350 ml, 3 feedings	A little	A little
31-60 days	400 ml, 2 feedings	100-150	Free choice
61-90 days	200 ml, 2 feedings	200-250	Free choice

d) **Mineral mixture**: the requirements of calcium and phosphorous for maintenance are 6.5 and 3.5 gm, respectively, per 50 kg body weight. Goats require slightly larger quantities of calcium than sheep. The mineral mixture may be included in the concentrate ration at the rate of 2 per cent.

e) **Salt:** Salt licks or lumps of rock salt of fairly good size should be hung up in some suitable place where the goats can easily get them. This is important as goats secrete a good amount of sodium and chloride ions in the milk.

f) **Vitamins and antibiotics:** Goats particularly need vitamins A, D and E. Vitamin A can be supplied by feeding green forage and yellow maize; 1 kg of lush-green fodder will provide 1500 IU. Vitamin D can be obtained by exposure to sunlight. Vitamin E is present in adequate amounts in most normal rations. Synthetic vitamins A and D may be supplemented in the ration of growing kids. Feeding of aureomycin or terramycin increases the growth rate of young kids, reduces the incidence of scours and other infectious diseases and also improve general appearance of kids.

Housing

Housing of goats is not a serious problem. It is enough if the goats are provided with a dry, comfortable, safe and secure place, free from worms, and affording protection from excessive heat and inclement weather. In Indian villages goats are mostly kept under widespread shady trees when the Climate is dry, provided the goats are safe from thieves and predatory animals such as wolves and panthers. The kids are kept under large inverted baskets until they are old enough to run along with their mothers. Males and females are generally-kept together.

It is worthwhile to design a cheap house for goats which may result in increased milk and meat production. Some kind of housing is necessary if herds of goats are maintained in cities and at organized farms; adequate space, proper ventilation, good drainage and plenty of light should be provided for while constructing houses. Successful goat dairying largely depends on the site where goats are kept. Goats do not thrive on marshy or swampy ground. Grazing areas should be free from pits and shallow pools, as contact parasitic infections arise mainly from such places.

'Lean-to' Type Shed

The cheapest form of building is the 'lean-to' type shed located against the side of an existing building. Such a shed for a family of two goats should be 1.5 m wide and 3.0 m long. This length provides 0.3 m for the manger and 1.2 m for the goats; the remaining 1.5 m space is sufficient for two milking does with a stub wall between them. The height nearest the wall should be 2.3 m and on the lower side 1.7 m giving a slope of 0.6 11) to the roof, which may be tiled or thatched. An open-framed window of good size on the lower side and an open-framed door should be provided. Arrangements for storing hay or dried feed can be made overhead.

The plan for a house varies with the climatic conditions and the type of flock to be sheltered. In dry climates with a rainfall of 50 to 75 cm a long shed open on the sides, little exposed to weather and built on well -drained ground makes an excellent shelter. A goat, when reared singly, can be housed in any building provided it is dry, free from draft and well ventilated. The space allowed should be 1.8 m x 1.8 m. A plain board, 28 cm wide and 2.5 cm thick with two circular holes sufficiently large for receiving two small galvanized iron pails, may be used in place of the manger or a trough for food. It should be raised 50 to 60 cm from the floor, supported on wooden or iron brackets fixed to the wall. These pails, one for water and the other for food, are preferred to the manger, as the accumulated residue of feed can be easily removed from them.

In the tropics because of high temperature, heavy rainfall and the susceptibility of goats-to parasitism, the most practical goat houses are those which are raised above the ground level, are well ventilated, and have long eaves to prevent heavy rain showers to splash in from the sides. The floor must be strong (wooden strips with small slits in between) and the roof material should provide effective insulation from the solar radiation. The roofing material would be made of bamboo or tree leaves or earthen tiles which are cheap and practical. Provision must be made for collection of dung and urine periodically.

Shelter for Buck

The buck should be housed separately. A single stall measuring 2.5 m x 2.0 m with the usual fittings for food and water would be suitable for the bucks. Two bucks should not be kept together, particularly during the breeding season, because they might fight.

Space for Goats in Stanchions and Confinement

The size of the stanchion where the goat is kept should be 0.75 m wide and 1.2 m long. Goats kept longer in a pen should have a floor space of 2 m^2.

Loose Stalls for Pregnant Does and Kids

Kids should be provided with separate loose stalls, away from adult females. The walls and doors of these stalls should be about 1.3 m high. A box barrel or a log is provided for exercise. One stall measuring 1.8 m^2 can accommodate up to 10 kids. Such loose stalls are also suitable for goats at the time of kidding. All stalls should be provided with an enclosure in which the animals can be let loose during the day. This loose housing system reduces the housing cost and labour.

Exercise Paddock for Stall-fed Goats

An enclosure measuring 12 m x 18 m is adequate for 100 to 125 goats. Such an enclosure or exercise paddock should be well fenced with strong woven wires which should not be far apart near the bottom. The exercise paddocks should be made bigger than the enclosures and should have some shade trees if the stock is to be maintained constantly in confinement. An extra-strong woven wire should be used, as goats have the habit of climbing fences and also of rubbing their bodies against them. Barbed wire should not be used so as to avoid injury to the udder and teats. It will be good if a box of 1 m x 1 m and 60 cm high and a stationary steel-drum or a log of 30 cm x 2.4 cm size is provided for their exercise.

Segregation Shed

When the herd is large, provision for a small segregation shed, about' 3·6 m x 5 m, is very desirable. It should be built in the farther comer of the farm and provided with a well-fenced yard; it should be divided into two or three sections. Each stall as well as the yard should have a' separate watering arrangement.

Recommended Floor and Trough Space for Goats in intensive Production Related to Live Weight:

	Weight	Floor Space			Trough Space
		Solid Floor	Slatted Floor	Open Yard	
	kg	m²/animal	m²/animal	m²/animal	m/animal
Doe	35	0.8	0.7	2	0.35
Doe	50	1.1	0.9	2.5	0.40
Doe	70	1.4	1.1	3	0.45
Kid	-	0.4 - 0.5	0.3 - 0.4	-	0.25 - 0.30
Buck	-	3.0	2.5	-	0.5

Tethering

When one or two goats are to be kept and facilities for grazing are limited, tethering is convenient. This simple device has the advantage of keeping goats out-of-doors, and at same time on a limited area, although frequent changes of location become necessary. The animal is provided with a shelter with in its reach so that it may turn to it in the event of extreme heat or heavy rains. Goats have strong dislike for rain and for getting wet. The shelter should be temporary and preferably a portable one. The rope or chain used for tethering should be about 35 to 50cm long. The peg should be tethered only in the morning and evening, and kept in the shed during the mid-day. Tethering has also an important advantage of grazing the animal on a plot which is definitely known to be free from parasitic infections.

Elevated Platform

In the tropics because of high temperature, heavy rainfall and the susceptibility of goats to parasitism, the most practical goat houses are those which are raised above the ground level, are well ventilated, and have long eaves to prevent heavy rain showers to splash in from the sides. The floor must be strong (wooden strips with small slits in between) and the roof material should provide effective insulation from the solar radiation. The roofing material would be made of bamboo or tree leaves or earthen tiles which are cheap and practical. Provision must be made for collection of dung and urine periodically.

Farming systems

1. Extensive System

- Grazing the sheep and goat in the entire pasture and leaving them there for the whole season is the extensive system of rearing.
- In this method feed cost is very much reduced.
- It is not conducive to make the best use of the whole grasses. So we can preferably practice the **rotational grazing method.**

Rotational grazing method

- Rotational grazing should be practiced under which the pasture land should be divided by temporary fences into several sections.

- The animals are then moved from one section to another section. By the time the entire pasture is grazed, the first section will have sufficient grass cover to provide second grazing.
- Parasitic infestations can be controlled to a great extent.
- Further, it helps to provide quality fodder for most part of the year.
- Under this system, it is advisable to graze the lambs first on a section and then bring in ewes to finish up the feed left by the lambs.

2. Semi-intensive system

- Semi-intensive system of sheep / goat production is an intermediate compromise between extensive and intensive system followed in some flocks having limited grazing.
- It involves extensive management but usually with controlled grazing of fenced pasture.
- It consists of provision of stall feeding, shelter at night under shed and 3 to 5 hour daily grazing and browsing on pasture and range.
- In this method, the feed cost is somewhat increased.

Advantages of this system

- Meeting the nutrient requirement both from grazing and stall feeding.
- Managing medium to large flock of 50 to 350 heads and above.
- Utilizing cultivated forage during lean period.
- Harvesting good crop of kids both for meat and milk.
- Making a profitable gain due to less labour input.

3. Intensive system-(zero grazing-system)

- It is a system in which sheep goats are continuously kept under housing in confinement with limited access in which they are stall fed.
- It implies a system where goats are not left to fend for themselves with only minimum care.

- Intensive operation of medium sized herd of 50 to 250 heads or more oriented towards commercial milk production goes well with this system particularly of dairy goats.
- It merits exploitation of the system of feeding agro-industrial by products as on fodder grass with carrying capacity of 37 to 45 goats per hectare.
- This system of management requires more labour and high cash input.
- However, this has the advantage of close supervision and control over the animals.
- In this method, the dung is collected in one place and used as a good fertilizer.
- Less space is sufficient for more number of animals.

5

Parasitic Diseases of Livestock and Their Sustainable Control

R. Katoch, R. Godara, Anish Yadav and Sanku Borkataki

Division of Veterinary Parasitology, Faculty of Veterinary Sciences & Animal Husbandry, SKUAST-Jammu-181102

The livestock play a significant role in generating gainful employment in rural areas, particularly among the landless and marginal farmers. The Jammu region of state of Jammu and Kashmir possesses a huge livestock population which is maintained under different management systems. The region has a vast diversity in agro-climatic conditions (comprising low altitude, middle altitude and high altitude), and animal husbandry and pasture management practices. Despite having huge livestock, the production potentials are very low. There are various factors related with low production and among them parasitic diseases rank very high. In the region, the animals generally follow open grazing system and pastoral system which are major contributing factors to predispose them to parasitic diseases. The animals generally suffer from sub-clinical infections without showing apparent clinical symptoms. In comparison to bacterial or viral diseases, they cause less mortality but high morbidity resulting into huge economic losses to the farmers in the form of low milk, wool and meat production, retarded growth, emaciation, lowered draught capabilities and reduced absorption of food nutrients (Soulsby, 1982; Chaudhri and Singh, 2003). The major parasitic diseases of the ruminants reported from the region are gastrointestinal nematodosis amphistomosis, fasciolosis, lung worm infection, Babesiosis, Anaplasmosis, myiasis and tick infestation (Yadav *et al.*, 2005; Khajuria, 2010; Nazeer, 2011; Khajuria *et al.*, 2013).

The major gastrointestinal worms in small ruminants are as follows:

Name of Nematode (Size)	Location	Important morphological feature	Pathogenesis	Symptom/lesions
Haemonchus contortus (10-30mm)	Abomasum	Asymmetrical dorsal lobe supported by a Y-shaped dorsal ray, Spine like cervical papillae, barber's pole	Blood sucking 0.05ml/worm/day	Anaemia, mucous membrane pale, abomasal mucosa swollen & have bite marks
Mecistocirrus digitatus (31-43mm)	Abomasum	Symmetrical dorsal lobe, spicules long & slender united almost whole length	Blood sucking	Anaemia, mucous membrane pale, abomasal mucosa swollen & have bite marks
Ostertagia spp (7.5-8.5mm)	Abomasum	Anterior extremity slightly inflated, transversally striated, rest of body 25-35 longitudinal ridges, an accessory bursal membrane situated on dorsal side	Mature differentiated cells (mucous, zymogenic, parietal) are replaced by undifferentiat-ed cells	High level of pepsinogen, bright green color diarrhea, 'Morocco leather' appearance of abomasums.
Trichostrongy-lus spp (4-8mm)	Abomasum and small intestine	Ventral notch near anterior extremity	Displacement & disruption of basement membrane leading to villous atrophy	Hypoalbuminaemia, emaciation, dark diarrheic feces, ring worm lesions.
Cooperia spp (4.5-9.0mm)	Small intestine rarely in abomasum	Cephalic swelling, the externodorsal usually arise from the base of dorsal stem	-do-	-do-
Bunostomum spp (12-26mm)	Small intestine (ileum, jejunum)	Buccal capsule ventral margin bears a pair of chitinous plates, asymmetrical dorsal lobe, right externodorsal ray rise higher up on dorsal stem	Blood sucking	Hydro thorax, fluid in peri-cardium, bottle jaw
Gaigeria pachyscelis (20-30mm)	Small intestine (duodenum)	Voluminous dorsal lobe	Blood sucking	Marked blood suckers, leading to death
Oesophagstomum columbianum (12-22mm)	Small & Large intestine	Cephalic vesicle, large cervical alae, cervical papillae	Nodule formation	Persistent diarrhea, dark green color feces contain mucus & sometime blood, ileum & colon studded with nodules
Trichuris ovis (35-80mm)	Caecum	Anterior part long and slender, posterior part thick, one spicule surrounded by protrusible sheath, vulva at beginning of wide part.	Blood feeders, tunneling mucosa, create pool of blood	Diarrhea, thickening of mucosa

Fasciolosis: It is caused by *Fasciola hepatica* in high altitudes and *Fasciola gigantic* in low altitude below 1200msl. In Indian sub continent *Lymnaea rufescens* and *L.accuminata* act as intermediate host. In sheep acute and chronic form of infection occurs whereas in cattle and buffaloes only chronic form occurs. It occurs post rains i.e. September to December majority of animals are positive in rain fed area. It is common in buffaloes due to its feeding on grasses located near water bodies. Sheep with acute infection die suddenly from hemorrhage and liver damage with the first evidence of a problem being sudden death. Majority sheep reluctant to move due to abdominal pain, reveals lethargy and reduced grazing activity. Blood oozes out from natural orifices. It has to be differentiated from anthrax. Post-mortem examination show ruptures of liver into small pieces, red color fluid in peritoneal cavity and immature flukes in cavity.

Chronic fasciolosis is the most common form of liver fluke infection in sheep, goats and cattle - and particularly in more resistant hosts, such as horses and pigs. It occurs when the parasites reach the bile ducts in the liver. The fluke ingests blood, which produces severe anaemia and chronic inflammation and enlargement of the bile ducts. The clinical signs develop slowly. The animals become increasingly anaemic, appetite is lowered, the mucous membranes of the mouth and eyes become pale and some animals develop oedema under the jaw ('bottle jaw'). Affected animals are reluctant to travel. In chronic cases sheep show poor body condition and poor fleece quality. The affected sheep may die in emaciated state when compounded with pregnancy and lactation. Wool falls in patches. Chronic fasciolosis is diagnosed by demonstration of fluke eggs in faecal samples. Faecal samples can be tested using the coproantigen ELISA test. Mature flukes are demonstrated in the bile ducts and gall bladder at necropsy

Control should be on a preventive rather than a curative basis. For effective control: Use strategic anthelmintic treatment (Triclabendazole), to reduce the number of fluke in the host and the number of fluke eggs in pasture; reduce the number of intermediate host snails (Physical, biological and chemical methods); manage fluke-prone areas, to reduce exposure to infection.

Paramphistomosis

Paramphistomosis of domestic ruminants is widely prevalent in India. It cause high death rates in calves, sheep and goats and indirect losses from debility and decreased milk yield in cows and buffaloes. They are widely prevalent in plain irrigated region and mid and high hills of Jammu region. Its outbreaks are seasonal confined to the post-monsoon and drier months of the year, i.e. late September to March/ April. In enzootic areas the early infection may be acquired by grazing on marshy areas or on pastures inundated during the preceding rainy season. The stall fed animals may pick up infection from fodder or imperfectly dried hay from the snail infested fields or pastures. Late outbreaks are due to grazing on vegetations surrounding ponds, pools, banks of river and canals and other water bodies infested with snails.

The morbidity and mortality rates of Paramphistomes are very high. The major species of Paramphistomes encountered in ruminants of Jammu region are Paramphistomum cervi, Gigantocotyle explanatum, Gastrothylax crumenifer, Fischoederius elongatus, F. cobboldi, and Carmyreius spp. The clinical paramphistomosis results from massive invasion of mucosa of duodenum and adjacent parts of the alimentary tract by immature paramphistomes following heavy intake of metacercariae. The immature paramphistomes draw a plug of mucosa into their suckers, thus produce lesions showing erosion and petechiae on the mucosa. The small intestine become hyperaemic and oedematous. In acute paramphistomosis major symptoms seen are oedema, anorexia and diarrhea. With the appearance of oedema the appetite of animal decreases and later it is completely lost however the animal generally show increased thirst and drink small quantities of water frequently and also keep its muzzle dipped in water for considerable time. Within a week of the appearance of oedema, the animal develops diarrhea. The feces become loose day by day and in last become watery and foetid. In chronic cases rectal hemorrhages may occur which results in presence of blood clots in the feces. In severe cases, especially in cattle the diarrhea is projectile and later sphincter control is completely lost and feces are passed involuntarily. The visible mucous membrane becomes pale and almost white. The disease generally follow acute phase which is 5-10 days in sheep and sub-acute of 10-20days in cattle and buffaloes. Generally emaciation and prostration precede death.

Diagnosis is made by the recovery of immature flukes in diarrheic feces, post-mortem, history of the area, and presence of immature stages in snails and eggs in feces.

Control

a) Therapeutic: Oxyclozanide @10-12mg/kg body wt., Rafoxanide @ 7.5mg/kg/body wt.

b) Control of intermediate host: manual, chemical and biological.

c) Control by management:

   1. Avoid grazing near low lying areas or water bodies
   2. Serve clean tap water for drinking to animals
   3. Fence/Dry out water bodies in pasture.
   4. Herbage from water bodies should be converted in to silage of hay before use.
   5. In paddy growing areas use of raw manure for fertilizing the fields results in high infection in snails and grass in these areas is heavily infested with metacercariae. Thus farmers should be educated.

Sustainable control of parasites

Worms means "Wisely thinking in opportunities and Resources available with us and their integration into formulation of Programme for parasite Management with the aim of Sustainability in production" (Singh and Swarnkar, 2011). Under extensive conditions follows in the region, only anthelmintic treatment will not provide sufficient control and there is a risk due to widespread occurrence of resistance to these chemicals. In addition, due to decrease in pasture land and increasing stringency of maximum permissible residue levels for meat and wool in export market has compelled to enhance search for other means of control (Newton, 1995). Under evasive strategies, following steps should be taken into consideration-

Knowledge of epidemiology

The prevalence of parasites depends upon agro-climatic conditions, animal husbandry practices and pasture management in a particular area. For example, *Paramphistomum* species are more prevalent in the low-lying canal irrigated areas of Jammu region (Yadav *et al.*, 2005; Khajuria *et al.*, 2013), whereas *Fasciola* species are mainly restricted to middle and high altitudes (Khajuria, 2010). However, gastrointestinal nematodes are found throughout the Jammu region. For better and appropriate control strategies, it is important to identify the epidemiological and ecological aspects of parasites and the associated risk factors that are unique to a particular area and farming system. Once the epidemiology is established, a control strategy can be implemented.

Improve nutritional status of the host

The presence of helminths, particularly in the digestive system causes decrease in food consumption, malabsorption and changes in host metabolism (Swarnkar and Singh, 2005). It has been reported that parasites have special affinity to vitamins and minerals such as the infection of *Diphyllobothrium latum* in man causes deficiency of vitamin-B12, leading to pernicious anaemia (Soulsby, 1982). Haemonchosis in small ruminants has a direct relationship with cobalt deficiency, as cobalt is used to synthesize vitamin B-12 and its deficiency further leads to internal parasitism (Katoch, 2005). Moreover, haemonchosis in small ruminants and hookworm infections in canines cause deficiency of iron and thus lead to anaemia (Lapage, 1959; Miller, 1971; Soulsby, 1982).

Manipulation of the host nutrition could represent an option to improve the host resistance. Vitamins A, D and B-complex are the important component of the diet to develop resistance against gastrointestinal helminths (Lapage, 1959). The increased protein supply in the diet increases the resistance of the host against helminths which resulted into reduced worm burden and suppression of growth and fecundity of worms (Molan *et al.*, 2000). Introduction of molasses/ mineral feed blocks and use of dewormer plus mineral mixture in the diet is recommended to improve the general nutrition of the animals as well-nourished animals are less susceptible to infections. Many studies have established the antiparasitic effects of some plant secondary compounds amongst which tannins, present in some legume forages or in woody plants are most important (Paolini and Hoste, 2003; Swarnkar *et al.*, 2009). Therefore, the feeding of traditional tree fodder in hills is recommended.

Strategic deworming

Reducing the use of dewormers and decreasing the resistance development to these dewormers is the need of hour. Anthelmintic treatment should be provided at the end of rains as the infective larvae on pastures are in abundant after rains. The use of anthelmintics during late winter months will kill the hypobiotic larvae and reduce the levels of infective larvae of strongyles on pastures during early summer months. Another treatment during early summer (March-April) will kill the overwintered larvae plus peri-parturient rise. The use of effective flukicides (triclabendazole or oxyclozanide) in autumn (September-October) and mid-summer (May-June) can reduce incidences of fasciolosis (in middle and high altitudes) and paramphistomosis (in low-lying areas) in Jammu region. Do not move animals to pasture immediately after deworming as all the dead worms with viable egg in them will contaminate the pasture. Again, changing the class of anthelmintic after some period will further reduces the risk of resistance development.

Judicious use of anthelmintics

Generally farmers like quick and easy solution and they think that controlling worms by management is more complicated than a standard treatment programme and therefore, a "treat and forget" approach seems to be preferable and there is a widespread use and misuse of anthelmintics. These frequent dosing results in development of anthelmintic resistance. Only those animals should be treated that get most benefit from the treatment, leaving the rest of the flock untreated.

Application of part-flock treatment

Sheep and goat flocks should be screened for anaemia by visual appearance of gradation in conjunctiva using colour chart and treat only those animals which are anaemic, particularly during wormy season.

Switching to herbal dewormers

Many herbs have now been evaluated for their antiparasitic activities. Plants like garlic and *Sericea lespedeza* works well against internal parasites. Sudden drop in fecal egg count due to tannin component of plants has been reported (Min, 2004).

Pasture management

Due to commercialization in last few decades, the pasture land is decreased while there is an increase in the animal population resulted into over stocking rate. Increased number of animals on the pastures will increase contamination of the pastures as well as the mass of herbage is reduced and infective larvae will be accessible more easily. The height of the pasture should be maintained greater than 2 inch and providing browsing area can reduce the parasitic load as larvae climbs up to one inch of height of grass blades. Beside the animals should be grazed in late morning hours, as it is well proven that after increasing in temperature the larvae move downwards and are not available on the upper parts of the grass blades.

During rainy and post rainy months, the contamination of pastures increased many folds (Katoch *et al.*, 1998; Sharma *et al.*, 2004; Yadav *et al.*, 2004), hence during this period the animals should be stall fed with the leaves of fodder tree or straw feeding should be provided. During summer months, the larvae remain at the lowest part, thus the animals are not allowed to graze very close to the ground. In addition, the pastures followed by crops should be preferred instead the pastures grown continuously. Further, avoiding grazing in wet patches of pasture and fencing off naturally wet areas reduces the infection rate. Furthermore, rotational grazing of sheep and goat with cattle and horse and providing tannin rich forage decrease the worm burden of animals.

Separation of young and adults

The young animals are more susceptible to parasitic infections than the adults (acquired age resistance). When young animals grazed with adults, they pick up infection in the early age and are the real sufferers.

For this "follower system" will be applied (in organised farms) in which young animals are grazed ahead of adults.

Selecting resistance animals

Breeding of selectively resistant animals is also helpful in decreasing the worm burden of ruminants. Selection at breed level and even individual level can contribute. These resistant animals also remain productive in parasitic contaminated environment.

Immunity

With the advancement of age, the animals usually develop some immunity against parasites. The animals that are poorly nourished, immunocompromised and young animals in which immune system has still not been developed are more prone to parasitic infections. So another way to reduce the production losses is to boost up the immunity level of animals. This can be done with vaccination, high plan of nutrition and using some compounds like copper oxide particles which has direct effect on internal parasites and also increases immunity (Singh and Swarnkar, 2011).

Interruption of life cycle

The life cycle of strongyle worms, especially *Haemonchus contortus* which have a short life span and majority of infective larvae disappearing from pasture within 4-6 weeks, can be broken either by adopting stall feeding (commercial flocks) for at least two months (implementation of cut and carry practice for fodder) or by adopting pasture resting strategy or rotational grazing.

Manure management

It is an effective method but cannot practice in our country and the animal faeces during grazing are the only manure they get (Katoch, 2005). Part of this is also collected by the poor people and used as fuel (dry pats).

Suggested Readings

1. Chaudhri, S.S. and Singh, D. (2003). Epidemiology of gastrointestinal nematodes in small ruminants. *In:* Helminthology in India (edited by M.L. Sood), International Book House, Dehradun.
2. Katoch, R. (1998). Epidemiological, chemotherapeutic and immunological studies on *Haemonchus contortus* of goats. Ph.D thesis submitted to CSAU of Agriculture and Technology, Kanpur.
3. Lapage, G. (1959). Monnig's Veterinary Helminthology and Entomology, 4th ed., Bailliere, Tindall and Cox, London, p 511.
4. Nazeer, T. (2011). Epidemiological and chemotherapeutic studies of parasites of buffalo. M.V.Sc thesis submitted to Sher-e-Kashmir University of Agricultural Sciences and Technology, Jammu.
5. Soulsby EJL (1982) Helminths, arthropods and protozoa of domesticated animals, 7th ed, Bailliere and Tindal, London, UK.

6

Feeds and Feeding of Dairy Animals

A.K. Pathak and Ankur Rastogi

Division of Animal Nutrition, Faculty of Veterinary Sciences & Animal Husbandry, SKUAST-Jammu-181102

Feeds and feeding of dairy animals are arguably the most important part of the dairy farm management. And it is not only what we feed that is important but how we manage our feeding is equally as critical. What we feed today not only determines the animal's milk production but also influences their entire lactation cycle that follows. Dairy animal feeding with balanced ration influences health status, reproductive, productive performance and better economic return in organic environment, all of which are critical to a profitable and sustainable dairy business as well as welfare of the dairy farmers. Feed costs currently account for around 45 percent of total milk price on average, with concentrates representing around 35 percent and forages around 10 percent. The range within this is substantial and there is a strong economic incentive to ensure that neither too little of a nutrient is given (limiting potential production or adding expenses through poorer health and fertility) nor too much, being wasteful.

The traditional feeding system for dairy animals is based on the use of poor quality crop residues like wheat straw, rice straw, sorghum and maize stovers, and natural grasses, supplemented with a little or no concentrates. The quantity and quality of fodder available from natural pasture shows seasonal fluctuation. There is an acute shortage of feed supply during off season and the available feed during this period is of very poor quality. Poor nutrition results in low production and reproductive performance, slow growth rate, loss of body condition and increased susceptibility to diseases and parasites. Thus, effective utilization of the available feed resources and appropriate supplementation of poor quality natural pasture and crop residue based diets appear to be the necessary steps to alleviate the nutritional problems of dairy animals. However, balanced feeds and better feeding management will have the biggest impact on dairy business performance. Therefore, perfect knowledge of dairy manager regarding dairy animal nutrition is essential in managing the high performance of dairy herd. It is more important, how that diet is fed and how the animals are managed will provide much greater variation in delivering nutrients to the animals with a significant impact on dairy farming.

The main motive of feeding dairy animals is to provide a balanced diet that allows the full potential genetic merit of the animal to be supported and milk production maximised, support both the health and fertility of dairy animals and the microbial population of their rumen and ensure that both of the above are done in the most economically efficient manner possible.

This is achieved by feeding a balance of energy sources, protein, fibre, starch and sugars and vitamins and minerals to a group of dairy animals. This balance of nutrients can be estimated with a reasonable degree of accuracy at a group level, and requirements met through the careful selection of appropriate locally available feed ingredients.

Nutrient such as proteins, carbohydrate fats, minerals, vitamins and water supplied through any feed constituent or group of constituents that are supported the life of all living being (organisms, animals and plants). Each type of nutrients has some special function to perform. All these nutrients provided to the animals which are coming from plants sources (feeds and fodders) and from animal products and their by-products, etc. The animal feeds are classified in two broad terms like roughage and concentrate.

Roughages

Roughages are bulky feeds containing relatively large amount of less digestible material i.e. crude fibre more than 18 percent and low in total digestible nutrients (TDN; less than 60 percent). Roughages are subdivided in to two major groups i.e. succulent and dry roughages based on the moisture content. Succulent feeds usually contain moisture from 60-90%, where as dry roughages contain only 10-15% moisture. For the sake of convenience succulent feeds are again classified into 'pastures, cultivated fodder crops, tree leaves, silage and root crops. Dry roughages are dried plant materials and or crop residues (wheat, paddy straw, maize and sorghum stovers), which are stored and/or preserved for usage in summer and in unforeseen climatic conditions.

Naturally grown grasses in the forest/ near railway track/ wastelands are rich in protein and highly palatable. It is better to feed in right growth stage. Pastures form the oldest form of livestock feed which allowed grazing to the animal. The word pastures refer to land on which different types of edible grasses and other plants grow or are grown for grazing livestock. Permanent pastures are those covered with perennial or self-seeding animal species of plants. Temporary pastures are those planted with quick growing crops like Sudan grasses and millet to provide supplemental grazing during lean season.

The cultivated fodder are the another source of good quality forages which are of two types i.e. leguminous and non-leguminous. Leguminous fodder consists of stem and leaves of a group of plants which contains 2-3% DCP and 10% TPN (such as cowpea, berseem, lucerne and sunhemp). Leguminous fodders are good source of protein, calcium, carotene but poor in phosphorus. For dairy animals (cattle and buffaloes), if legumes are fed *ad-lib*, there is no need for any additional supply of protein. But sometimes it may cause frothy bloat and reproductive disorders in dairy animals if we fed in large amounts for longer duration due to presence of saponine and estrogenic substances, respectively.

Non-leguminous fodders (0.5-1 percent DCP and 10-15 percent TDN) consists of many cereal crops (maize, sorghum, MP Chari, bajra), cultivated grasses (Paragrass, Napier grass), indigenous grasses (Dhub grass) and introduced grasses (Orchard grasses and Jungle/ Forest grasses). Certain fodder tree leaves are fed either in fresh form or tree leaf meal/ leaf meal mixture whenever fodder crisis occurs. Now days dried leaf meal or leaf meal mixture (Shahtoot, Subabul, Guava, Jamun, Babool, etc.) may also be supplemented in the diet as alternate feed resources. If the surplus green fodders are available in the season then they can be conserved in suitable form either in hay or silage.

The green crops when become mature and before formation of seeds are cut and air dried to reduce the moisture content to 15 percent to inhibit the enzyme which spoils the grass are known as hay. It may be leguminous or non-leguminous. Under leguminous Lucerne is best suitable crop for hay making. Lucerne hay contains 14-16% DCP and 50% TDN, while in non-leguminous fodder crops, oat hay is of better quality than other non-leguminous hay. Non leguminous hay is less palatable and contains lesser proteins than legume.

Poor quality crop residues are the stem parts of food crops after harvesting the cereals and grains are dried and known as straws like wheat and paddy straws, maize, sorghum stovers and kadbi, etc. Straws are poorest in protein and have largest percentage of crude fibre. They are comparatively poor in phosphorus, but rich in silica and oxalates. The straws contain DCP zero percent and TDN 40 percent.

Concentrate

A balanced concentrate mixture is a feed or feed mixture which supplies primary nutrient (proteins, carbohydrates and fat) at higher levels but contains less than 18% crude fibre and more than 60% TDN. Concentrates are classified as energy and protein rich concentrates. The crude protein will be less than 18% in energy rich concentrates. And more than 18% in protein rich concentrates. Cereals (locally available maize, barley, wheat, bajra, rice, sorghum, oats and bajra, etc) and their by-products (wheat bran, rice bran, de-oiled rice bran, gram husk, chunies and broken rice, etc) and other industries by-products (molasses), etc. comes under the categories of energy concentrates while the by-products after removing oils of oil seeds are important plant protein supplements (which contain more than 20 percent protein) like oil seed cakes (i.e. Ground nut, cotton seed, linseed, mustard, sunflower, soybean and til cake). The by-product of wine industry such as barley sprout and maize gluten also comes under the category of alternate protein source for ruminants feeding.

Many microbial feed additives for calf and dairy animals have been used which include bacterial cultures from both ruminal and non-ruminal sources. Most commonly used products are based on *Lactobacillus* spp., *Bifidobacterium* spp., *Aspergillus oryzae* and *Saccharomyces cerevisiae.* Supplementation of these probiotics and/or direct fed microbials (DFM) increased body weight gain, health status, immunity in young calves and milk yield to about 5-7% in dairy animals.

Water is one of the important nutrients which cannot be ignored and also an important source of minerals. Therefore, the mineral content of the water supply should be considered with regard to the total intake of dietary minerals. Depending on the quality of water supply available, water intake may make a substantial contribution to daily mineral intake, particularly with regard to sulphur and, in some areas of the country, salt. The most important factor which affects the animal performance is the intake and palatability of feed.

Feed intake

Feed intake is essentially the industry standard method of assessing how much a cow, or group of cows, is consuming at a particular point in their lactation cycle. It refers to the weight of feed consumed once all water has been removed - essentially the nutrients capable of being used for biological processes such as milk production and reproduction. The link between feed intake and production is easy to appreciate, and from a production standpoint it is one of the critical components of maximising milk and financial efficiency.

The implications of maximising feed intake, however, go far beyond milk production. Minimising the drop in feed intake around calving and maximising feed intake throughout lactation is the cornerstone of managing the early lactation energy deficit, which in turn has great bearing on whether an animal goes on to develop a metabolic disease, get in calf and ultimately whether she will reach the end of her lactation alive. When rationing for dairy cattle, promoting dry matter intake is critical as it will define which ingredients need to be selected in what proportions to meet cattle's requirements.

Dairy animals have a highly developed sense of taste and smell, and will readily reject feed they deem unpalatable if the opportunity is made available to them. They are also creatures of habit and generally prefer their feed to remain unvaried; this is unsurprising given their dependence on a very delicately balanced flora of rumen bacteria, fungi and protozoa that react slowly to dietary changes.

The composition of the ration, regardless of the ingredient quality, also has a bearing on palatability and therefore feed intake: some ingredients taste better than others. For example, feeding high inclusions of magnesium chloride to dry cows will stop milk fever, but may predispose to other problems as cows are reluctant to eat the ration due to the bitter taste.

The method of delivery of the ration is also important; greater intakes are afforded when a more natural method of feeding is followed, such as a mixed ration.

Feed formulation

The balanced ration should be formulated and updated regularly to avoid under and overfeeding of nutrients or fluctuations in milk production. The most common guideline for diet formulation is the available feeding standards in our country like BIS and ICAR feeding standards for dairy animals. These publications provide equations to compute nutrient requirements for any size animals and milk production level and any stage of the life cycle. Therefore, actual feed intakes can be determined that can help to formulate diets. Because of the complexity of formulating feeds to optimize production while minimizing excretion, producers not trained in nutrition should obtain help from qualified nutritionists when formulating diets.

Different supplementation strategies could be applied depending upon the type, accessibility and price of supplementary feeds in a given area. Now day's varieties of ways have been devised by farmers and their advisors to feed dairy animals which can be broadly given below:

Separate roughage and concentrate feeding

It is a simple system that allows tight allocation of supplementary feed and hence very good cost control and control of BCS in late lactation. Locally available cereal grains, grain by-products and cake are usually fed to produce milk but the amount of concentrate can be fed depends upon the milk yield and on stage of lactation or just flat rate fed. Care must be taken not to over feed in early lactation so cake allocations usually limited in first few weeks.

Concentrate supplementation

The balanced concentrate should be supplemented in the diet of dairy animals when they fed poor quality roughage. Its supplementation increases straws intake by 10-20 percent and improved nutrient utilization. Small amounts of specific protein supplements provide constant supply of nutrients to rumen microbes and thereby improve production performance of animals. Its supplementation provides adequate energy and nitrogen to the microbes along with essential minerals in a desirable proportion. Proportion of concentrate in the roughage based diet will also depend on the production level of the animal.

Minerals and vitamins supplementation

Available mineral mixture (with and without salt) as per BIS should be incorporated in the ration of dairy animals @ 2 percent (without salt) and 3 percent (with common salt). Calcium deficiency in young calves prevents normal bone growth and retards their general growth and development. In dairy animals with milk fever, uterus returns to normal size more slowly after calving and increases the incidence of dystocia, retained placenta and prolapsed uterus. Ratio of Ca: P in milking animal diets should be kept between 1.5 to 2.5, however, one must remember that the amount of each of these minerals is more important than Ca to P ratio. A deficiency of trace minerals like Cu, Zn, I, Mn and Co in the diet of dairy animals may depress the reproductive performance.

Vitamin A, D and E are very much essential for all physiological stages of animals like growth, reproduction and production. Retarded growth, reproductive problems associated with a vitamin A deficiency include delayed sexual maturity, abortion, and birth of dead or weak calves, retained placenta, metritis and shortened gestation periods. Supplementation of vitamin A should be considered when feeding poor quality forages or low amounts of forage and corn silage. Beta-carotene is a precursor of vitamin A. Reproductive performance can be improves when animal supplemented with beta-carotene. Vitamin D is necessary for normal calcium and phosphorus metabolism and thus, affects reproduction indirectly. Vitamin E and selenium have been used successfully in combination to reduce the incidence of retained placenta, metritis and cystic ovaries in herds having low level of these nutrients. Supplementation of pregnant cattle and buffaloes with 1000 IU of vitamin E during last 60 days of pregnancy till 30 days post parturition controls the problems of mastitis.

Partial mixed ration feeding

The most common system used in the country. Concentrate or oil cakes are fed either in parlour or out-of-parlour and a mixed ration fed in troughs etc. The mixed ration can be as simple as top-dressing the forage supply with a straight or compound feed; it is a blend of forages and supplementary feeds in a mixer wagon. Many, many variants exist with one or more mixed rations fed in the trough, and various ways of allocating the supplementary feed based on stage of lactation, milk yield or flat rate, or flat rate to one or more groups. Can be very flexible and cost effective in terms of feed use but often has the highest capital costs.

Total mixed ration (TMR) feeding

All feedstuffs like balanced concentrate mixture, dry roughage, green fodders and other feed supplements should be mixed together in the feed mixer and fed out down the trough with no individually allocated supplementary feed. Its feeding works well for bigger herds and higher yields. Savings can be made from buying straights direct but need to buy and store one or more 29T tipped loads to get best savings so some will use simple blends. Needs care and time to prepare and feed out the TMR which can become a major demand in complex systems. In its purest form the entire milking herd fed one standard TMR works well for high yielding herds with good fertility when the lactation and feed intake curves are similar.

Densified complete feed block feeding

It is intimate mixture of processed roughages, balanced concentrate mixture, other supplementary nutrients and bypass nutrients in a compressed desirable form and proportions capable to fulfil nutrient requirement of dairy animals. The feeding of densified complete feed blocks stabilizes rumen fermentation, minimizes fermentation loss and ensures better ammonia utilization. This pattern of rumen fermentation enhances utilization of poor quality roughage and improves the palatability of unconventional feeds. Because of seasonal availability and low bulk density, storage, handling and transportation of roughage materials become very difficult. Thus, complete feed in block form may overcome the above problem and will transport feed resources to deficit region or area of natural calamities cost effectively and can form a part of scarcity feed banks for economic and viable animal production programmes for small and marginal farmers, landless labourers and other weaker sections of the society as well as dairy farms of nearby cities. Their feeding improve growth rate (30-40%) i.e. @ 600-800 g/ day, milk yield up by 10-15 %, brings consistency with peak persistency, improves health and reproductive performance , reduces treatment cost, labor cost on feeding by 30%, easy to handle, to store, and to feed. Their feeding also reduces feed wastage, clean mangers, avoid selective feeding and overall cost effective and environment friendly technology.

Urea molasses multi nutrient blocks supplementation

Urea molasses multi nutrient blocks are the readymade supplements for dairy animals which contain all nutrients like carbohydrates, fats, protein, non-protein nitrogenous substances (urea), all essential major and trace minerals, vitamins and other feed additives in a balanced proportion to fulfil the need of ruminants which are basically reared on poor quality sub-maintenance type of roughage. The principles for improving the use of poor quality roughages by dairy animals include supplementation of fermentable nitrogen, soluble carbohydrates source and minerals which could bypass the rumen and this could be in form of multi nutrient blocks. These blocks should contain all essential nutrients in balanced proportion that could be made from a variety of feed ingredients depending on their local availability, nutritive value, price, existing facilities for their use and their influence on the quality. These are basically concentrated form of lick blocks by which animals can licks according to their nutritional needs.

Dietary supplementation of urea molasses multi nutrient blocks in the ration of dairy animals improves the digestion and utilization of nutrients. It is effective in increasing nutrient digestibility of low quality roughages improve ruminal fibre digestion. Its feeding improve rumen ecosystem which is beneficial to rumen microbial activity, and hence rumen digestion. Their supplementations also improve growth, health status, and reproductive performance and optimize production potential of dairy animals. Their supplementation @ 400-500 g/animal/day increased milk yield 1-1.5 kg/animal/day, better reproductive performance and lower inter calving period when fed straw based diets.

Importance of feeding

Feeding of calf

Feeding of colostrum to newly born calf after birth within 1-2 hours to get maximum antibodies for developing immunity against diseases. Biological significance of the colostrum will be lost if feeding is delayed for more than 2 hours. Dairy animals in 2nd or later lactation's produce larger quantity of colostrum and have higher immunoglobulins concentrations than animals in first lactation. This is because old animals would have been exposed to a wider range of diseases than young animals and therefore have produced more immunoglobulins against them. The calf is capable of absorbing antibodies from the colostrum only for a short period of time. It should be fed @ 1/10th of calf body weight. Maximum absorption of immunoglobulin as such occurs immediately after birth due to the process of pinocytosis and decrease with time because 24 hours after birth immunoglobulins degraded in the intestine.

Calves should be fed according to their weight. They require 1 kg milk for every 10 to 12 kg body weight per day. The calf's appetite and condition may also be taken into account. Rate of growth and age are other important factors. After 4-5 fays calf should be fed whole milk @ one tenth of calf s body weight. It can be replaced by skim milk at a gradient rate. Skim milk feeding may be discontinued at 24 weeks of age. Normal butter milk or reconstituted skim milk also is fed in place of fresh skim milk for raising dairy calves especially when calves have access to legume hay.

After 4 months of age, calf can utilize grain mixture. The amount of grains needed for calf will depend upon the quality of roughages. Clean, green and leafy legume or mixed hay forms the good fodder for young calves, hay can be offered to young calves after two weeks of age on free choice basis. They may start with handful of hay but will eat more and more with increase in age. Green legumes preferable mixed with other fodder are also good. Pasture specially a mixture of legume with other grasses provides an excellent, feed for growing calves. They may be permitted to graze after 6 months of age. A separate pasture for calves is suggested. A limited quantity of silage may be offered to calves preferably after 4 months of age. Care should be taken only 3-4 kg good quality silage along with mineral supplements.

Calves should have an abundant supply of minerals particularly calcium and phosphorus. The requirement of these minerals is partly met when legume hay it fed liberally. A simple mineral mixture consisting of 2 parts of dicalcium phosphate and one part salt will usually give results. In areas where deficiency of Iodine and cobalt exists, the iodised salt and cobalt chloride should be included in mineral mixture. When the amount of whole milk in the diet of calf is being limited, the Vitamin A and D should be supplied in calf starter. Sun cured hay is also a good source of Vitamin D calves receiving available sunshine probably do not lack Vitamin D. Rovimix can also be added as a good source of Vitamin A, B2 and D.

Growing calves should have free access to fresh, clean water at all times, particularly when milk feeding is reduced. Heifer is growing animals and so the requirements for growth is of higher order than for more maintenance during early stage relatively more protein is required than energy. Most young heifers grow well if excellent hay is given as much as they eat. The amount of growth depends upon the quality of forage in unlimited amounts. No grains need to be fed after the calf is 9 months. Feed *adlib* of green fodder so that the animal gets enough carotene. If leguminous fodders are fed it gives enough calcium, and other minerals. When the heifers are fed with *adlib* roughages and concentrates and then check for their growth. If only poor quality crop residues are fed then they should be supplemented with multi nutrient blocks for obtaining proper body weight gain and early maturity in growing heifers.

Feeding of pregnant and lactating animals

If the pregnant and lactating animals are fed liberally with good quality green fodder, vitamin A supplementation should be stopped.

Basal diet should not be restricted as a rule of thumb; 3 g of fermentable nitrogen per 100 g of fermentable organic matter are required to meet the needs for efficient microbial growth. Feeding of 30-40 grams of mineral and vitamin supplements per animal per day may be beneficial in urea treated straw based diet. In pregnancy, feed intake is low (about 1.7- 2% of body weight). Pregnant dry animals (more than 5 month of pregnancy) should be fed with 20-30 Kg green fodder and 1-2 Kg concentrate mixture (20% CP and 70% TDN) and *ad libitum* wheat straw, respectively.

It has been shown that in last tri-master of pregnancy, pregnant heifers need an extra 0.5 kg balanced concentrate mixture per day, in addition to its maintenance requirements. During the last trimester of pregnancy, a further quantity of 1.25 and 1.75 kg balanced concentrate mixture is recommended for cattle and crossbred cattle/ buffaloes, respectively. During last tri-master (advance stage) of pregnancy an additional amount 90 to 130 g of DCP and 1-1.1 kg TDN have to be provided to cattle and buffaloes of 350 kg to 500 kg body weight. During the last 3 days prior to calving, the amount of concentrate mixture should be reduced and a little warm bran is fed to keep the animal in laxative condition before calving.

Dietary manipulation is the alteration of the roughage to concentrate ratio during lactation and during dry period. Forage to concentrate ratio regulate the metabolic activity of dairy animals and determines whether they should be in a state to produce milk or to fatten efficiently. When diets exceed 60 percent concentrate on a dry matter bases, rumen pH was depressed and the animals' metabolic activity shifted from milk production to body weight gain and fattening.

The two concepts can be implemented by feeding a combination of non-protein nitrogen (NPN) compounds like urea, minerals, vitamins, soluble carbohydrates and by-pass protein. By-pass protein is relatively new concept which suggests that milk production, once the efficiency of utilisation of the basal feed resource has been optimised, depends upon providing nutrients needed for the components of milk, e.g. the quantity and balance of glucose (for milk lactose), protein and fat, in a form that will by-pass the rumen.

In high yielding animals about 8 percent of the total protein requirement should be in the form of bypass protein (protected protein/ rumen un-degradable protein). Feeding of high milk yielders with high plane of nutrition there is depression in the digestibility of feed. To overcome these problems, 3 percent extra rations may be given for each 10 litres of milk produced above 20 kg and the feeding frequency of the ration may be increased. To allow for growth of young lactating animals, increase the maintenance allowances for all nutrients except vitamin A and D by 20 percent during 1st lactation and 10 percent during 2nd lactation.

In practice, a mixture of concentrates (CP 20-22% and TDN 70-72%) is prepared by using locally available feed ingredients in different proportions like grains (maize, wheat, jowar and bajra in30-33%), cereal by-products (wheat bran, rice bran, de-oiled rice bran, pulse chunies, broken rice, rice husk and gram husk, 30-33%), and Molasses (5-10%), and Urea (1%), oil cakes viz. cotton seed cake, mustard cake, ground nut cake, soybean meal, sunflower cake, etc. (25-32%), mineral mixture (1.5 - 2%) and common salt (1-1.5%). To fulfil their vitamin needs locally available green fodder (leguminous and non-leguminous) and for providing bulk, dry roughages viz. wheat straw, paddy straw, kadbi, etc. were fed the animals. Grains and concentrate should be fed only to meet additional requirements such as growth, pregnancy and milk production and the coefficient of digestion is 5-8% higher in buffaloes than in cattle.

Supplementation with tree leaves as natural protein protectants usually is the most economical way. Supplementation with bypass oil is also beneficial especially for milk production and growth since this can be incorporated directly into milk and body fat and is less costly. On high fibre diets, unprotected fat added above 5 percent of the diet DM depress fibre digestion. If the poor quality roughages are surplus and it is the sole source of diet, problems in balancing the nutrients to dairy animals then they should go for multi nutrient block supplementation or feeding of total mixed ration and achieve and maintain production performance up to their genetic potential. If the scarcity/ deficiency good quality feed and fodders, problems in handling, storage and procurement of different feedstuffs from local market then they should be advised to feed their animals with densified complete feed blocks.

Feeding of dairy animals during transition period and stress conditions

Feeding of transition animals with forage and concentrate, as a TMR should be encouraged to ensure forage to grain ratio remains constant. Maximizing feed intake during the transition period must be a priority. Provide high quality forages and avoid sudden changes in diet ingredients. Avoid unnecessary stress near the time of calving. Feeding extra concentrate during the final 2 to 3 weeks prior to calving would benefit animal by adopting rumen to high starch diets and providing additional energy during a period when feed intake normally declines. Energy is one of the most important limiting factors in the synthesis of milk by the mammary gland. Inadequate availability of feeds during adverse climate affects the production performance of animals.

Heat stress reduces feed intake and increases water intake, causing a rapid decline in milk yield. Heat stress not only reduce feed intake, milk yield, but also results in decline of milk fat and solid not fat. An ambient temperature of above 40^{0}C depresses feed intake leading to mobilization of body reserves and high losses in body weight. In summer, the feed should be offered in the early morning and late evening so that animals feed intake and their milk production would be maintained. Both heat and cold stress increases the animals' maintenance requirement. However, cold stress increases feed intake, which prevents a decline in milk yield until temperature go below -5^{0}C. In hot-dry and hot-humid season feeding of total mixed ration (TMR) and/or densified complete feed blocks should be practiced to stop the decline in feed intake which helps in sustainment of milk production.

Good quality and sufficient quantity of feed and fodders and appropriate feeding is the cardinal feature in dairy animal production as the feed costs account for over half of the total milk production, increasing self sufficiency in feed production will be an important factor in future development programs. It is fundamental approach to provide good quality feed and fodders and/or balanced complete feed to dairy animals in sufficient amount to maximize production. The quality and quantity of feed that is utilized for milk production should be optimum to increase the profitability of dairy farmers. This is perceived to be difficult as the dairy animals are often a poor converter. As the utilization of dietary protein in the ruminant animals is lower than simple stomach animals because the digestion in ruminant animals depends essentially upon a fermentative process in rumen before the enzymatic digestion. The condition becomes more complex when the availability of feeds is scarce. In such situation the feeding strategy must aim at optimising rumen fermentation to obtain maximum nutrients from the forage based diets and supplementation with nutrients at the intestine by bypassing the rumen fermentation to ensure the most favourable balance and efficiency on the use of the nutrients absorbed.

7

Small Scale Projects and Prospects of Small Ruminant Farming

Pranav Kumar

Assistant Professor, Division of Veterinary & Animal Husbandry Extension Education, Faculty of Veterinary Sciences & Animal Husbandry SKUAST-Jammu-181102

Small ruminants is a composite term used for sheep and goats. Throughout the developing countries, small ruminants make a very valuable contribution, especially to the poor in the rural areas. These contributions range from precious animal proteins (meat and milk) to fibre and skins, draught power in the highlands, food security and stable households. By and large, the importance and extent of the contributions are inadequately understood as a consequence of which these valuable genetic resources continue to be generally neglected. Research and development investments to improve the relatively low level of contribution do not match their potential importance, the contribution to nutritional security and livelihoods of the poor in rural areas. Species like goat and sheep are of short-generation interval, have a high prolificacy rate and require less land, investment and operational expenses and are better suited to the resource endowment of the poor. In India, small ruminants provide much needed livelihood support to the landless and weaker sections and hold considerable potential for commercialization. A stable sheep population in the last two decades produced around 40 million kg wool annually, of which only 4 million kg is of fine quality. Goat population grew faster than any other species of livestock and has been a major source of meat. Shrinking and degrading pastures coupled with limitations of fodder, Lack of sufficient veterinary care and apathy to assisted reproductive technologies have been the major constraints.

Importance of Small Ruminant Farming

Goat Farming

Why do goat rearing

Goat is a multi functional animal and plays a significant role in the economy and nutrition of landless, small and marginal farmers in the country. Goat rearing is an enterprise which has been practiced by a large section of population in rural areas. Goats can efficiently survive on available shrubs and trees in adverse harsh environment in low fertility lands where no other crop can be grown. In pastoral and agricultural subsistence societies in India, goats are kept as a source of additional income and as an insurance against disaster. Goats are also used in ceremonial feastings and for the payment of social dues. In addition to this, goat has religious and ritualistic importance in many societies. The advantages of goat rearing are:

i) The initial investment needed for goat farming is low.

ii) Due to small body size and docile nature, housing requirements and managemental problems with goats are less.

iii) Goats are friendly animals and enjoy being with the people.

iv) Goats are prolific breeders and achieve sexual maturity at the age of 10-12 months gestation period in goats is short and at the age of 16-17 months it starts giving milk. Twinning is very common and triplets and quadruplets are rare.

v) In drought prone areas risk of goat farming is very much less as compared to other livestock species.

vi) Unlike large animals in commercial farm conditions both male and female goats have equal value.

vii) Goats are ideal for mixed species grazing. The animal can thrive well on wide variety of thorny bushes, weeds, crop residues, agricultural by-products unsuitable for human consumption.

viii) Under proper management, goats can improve and maintain grazing land and reduce bush encroachment (biological control) without causing harm to the environment.

ix) No religious taboo against goat slaughter and meat consumption prevalent in the country.

x) Slaughter and dressing operation and meat disposal can be carried without much environmental problems.

xi) The goat meat is more lean (low cholesterol) and relatively good for people who prefer low energy diet especially in summer and sometimes goat meat (chevon) is preferred over mutton because of its "chewability"

xii) Goat milk is easy to digest than cow milk because of small fat globules and is naturally homogenized. Goat milk is said to play a role in improving appetite and digestive efficiency. Goat milk is non allergic as compared to cow milk and it has anti-fungal and anti bacterial properties and can be used for treating uro-genital diseases of fungal origin.

xiii) Goats are 2.5 times more economical than sheep on free range grazing under semi arid conditions.

xiv) Goat creates employment to the rural poor besides effectively utilising unpaid family labour. There is ample scope for establishing cottage industries based on goat meat and milk products and value addition to skin and fibre.

xv) Goat is termed as walking refrigerator for the storage of milk and can be milked number of times in a day.

Sheep Farming

Why Sheep Farming

Sheep with its multi-facet utility for wool, meat, milk, skins and manure, form an important component of rural economy particularly in the arid, semi-arid and mountainous areas of the country. It provides a dependable source of income to the shepherds through sale of wool and animals. The advantages of sheep farming are:

i) Sheep do not need expensive buildings to house them and on the other hand require less labor than other kinds of livestock.

ii) The foundation stock is relatively cheap and the flock can be multiplied rapidly.

iii) Sheep are economical converter of grass into meat and wool.

iv) Sheep will eat varied kinds of plants compared to other kind of livestock. This makes them excellent weed destroyer.

v) Unlike goats, sheep hardly damage any tree.

vi) The production of wool, meat and manure provides three different sources of income to the shepherd.

vii) The structure of their lips helps them to clean grains lost at harvest time and thus convert waste feed into profitable products.

viii) Mutton is one kind of meat towards, which there is no prejudice by any community in India and further development of superior breeds for mutton production will have a great scope in the developing economy of India.

Present status and trends

The small ruminants provide livelihood support to the poor underprivileged landless, and marginal farm households. The goat and sheep production systems are mainly subsistence-oriented but in view of the rising demand for meat, there is a great scope for their commercialization. Nonetheless, these animals have been grossly neglected in development programs and their potential for enhancing livestock growth remains untapped. India ranks 3rd in sheep population, next to China and Australia and is placed at the 7th position among the top 10 countries of the world in terms of mutton and wool production. Development of sheep has been at crossroads. The population of sheep has stagnated except a marginal increase between 2003 and 2007. The wool production has declined to around 40 million kg, of which fine wool is only 10%. The trade policy of permitting import of wool under OGL has affected domestic traditional market. A clear cut policy direction is needed on priority as to whether the focus should continue to raise sheep for wool production or the focus should shift towards mutton production. With as many as 42 descript breeds, Indian sheep wealth is valued at Rs.3600 crores and development of this species needs focused attention during 12th plan period and beyond.

Goat is one of main species for meat in India. It has all the characteristics required for efficient meat production viz. high prolificacy, more than one breeding season in a year, higher milk production and capacity to bear twins and triplets. Goat meat is preferred and fetches higher prices in national and international markets. In spite of the prejudice against goat rearing due to environmental issues, the population of this species has grown at a faster rate than any other species of livestock. The potential of raising Pashmina goats viz. Changthangi in Ladakh (J&K) and Chegu in higher altitudes in Himachal Pradesh for production of pashmina fibre has remained underexploited. The traditional transhumance system of rearing of sheep and goats with established migratory routes are becoming economically unviable and slowly waning due to several reasons.

The major limiting factors in improving sheep and goat production are lack of pastures and fodder shrubs and trees in the area where the sheep and goat abound, especially in the states of Rajasthan and the whole of the northern hill region. All efforts for improving high altitude pastures through aerial re-seeding with perennial temperate grasses and legumes have not been very successful. The higher stocking rates, excessive grazing pressure, change in plant composition of grazing areas and reduced biomass availability have rendered migratory system of rearing difficult to sustain. Excessive parasitic load in migratory flock, higher energy spent while covering greater distance during migration along with other factors lead to body weight loss resulting into poor remunerative price realization by migratory shepherd community.

A Report on Small Ruminant Husbandry in Jammu & Kashmir

Economic Analysis

During the year 2011-12 the total wool production estimated for the State was 75.295 Lakh Kg which consisted of 61.586 Lakh Kg (81.79%) from Cross-breed Sheep and 13.709 Lakh Kg (18.20%) of Local-breed Sheep. During the year 2010-11, the total wool production estimated for the state was 73.819 Lakh Kg. Meat production registered a growth from 308.986 Lakh Kg to 322.781 Lakh Kg in the year 2011-12 over the previous year resulting into 4.47% growth. During 2012-13, 10.88 million meters of handloom fabrics valuing Rs 246.97 Crore were produced in the cooperative sector.

There are 2040 handloom units in the State which provide employment to 2875 persons. These units are producing Loies, Puttos, Tweed, Blankets, Raffal, Pashmina and Dusoti Khad. The Department has 523 registered Handloom Industrial Co-operative Societies in the State with a membership of 15275 weavers. There are approximately 38,000 Handlooms in the State.

Estimated Region-wise Livestock Population for the year 2011-12 in J&K State (Population in Lakhs)

Item	Livestock Population (2011 – 12)			
	Kashmir Region	Jammu Region	Ladakh Region	Total
Sheep	16.261	20.812	2.131	**39.204**
Cross Bred	13.439	14.505	1.027	28.971
Local	2.882	6.307	1.104	10.293
Goat	3.172	12.054	2.91	**18.136**

Wool Production

- Average wool yield per annum is 26.218 Kg for cross-breed sheep and 17.495 Kg for local-breed sheep.
- During the year 2011-12 the total wool production estimated for the State was 75.295 Lakh Kg which consisted of 61.586 Lakh Kg (81.79%) from Crossbreed Sheep and 13.709 Lakh Kg (18.20%) of Local-breed Sheep. During the year 2010-11, the total wool production estimated for the state was 73.819 Lakh Kg.
- Total availability of wool per person per annum is 629.978 g for the state as a whole which included 515.278 g from Cross-breed Sheep and 114.700 g from Local-breed Sheep.

Meat Production

- As per the Integrated Sample Survey Report (ISS), 2011-12, total estimated meat production of State was worked out to be 322.781 Lakh Kg consisting of 80.79% of (260.762 Lakh Kg) Red Meat and 19.21% (62.019 Lakh Kg) of White Meat. As per the latest Integrated Sample Survey Report (ISS), 2010-11, total estimated meat production of State was worked out to be 308.986 Lakh Kg.
- As per estimated results of ISS survey 2011-12, the meat availability was worked out to be 2.701 Kg per person per year against 2.650 Kg for 2010-11.
- Meat production registered a growth from 308.986 Lakh Kg to 322.781 Lakh Kg in the year 2011-12 over the previous year resulting into 4.47% growth.

Trends of sheep and goat production in Jammu & Kashmir (Population in Lakh)

Division	Population
Jammu	39.07
Kashmir	21.68
Ladakh	6.39
Total	**67.14**

Population of sheep and goat in India

Sheep 65.06 million

Goat 135.17 million

Percentage share of J&K in sheep population: 5.71%

Percentage share of J&K in goat population: 0.14%

Sheep breeding farms in Kashmir & Ladakh

District	Location of Breeding Farms
Srinagar	Sheep Breeding Farm Dachigam
Budgam	Sheep Breeding Farm Kralpathri
Anantnag	Sheep Breeding Farm Daksum
Baramulla	Sheep Breeding Farm Hardshiva
Kupwara	Sheep Breeding Farm Poshnar
Kulgam	Sheep Breeding Farm Kewa
Bandipora	Goat Farm, Arin
Ganderbal	Sheep Breeding Farm Goabal
Shopian	Sheep Breeding Farm Zawoora
Leh	i. Russian Merino Sheep Farm Mathoo ii. Pashmina Goat farm Upshi iii. Pashmina Goat farm Khuril, Neyoma iv. Dairy Goat Farm Hunder v. Mohair Goat Farm Satakna
Kargil	i. Merino Sheep Farm Lakthang ii. Karakul Sheep Farm Khumbathang iii. Pashmina Goat Farm Khangrial iv. Angora Goat Farm Pashkun Mathoo

Infrastructure Available With Sheep Husbandry, Jammu

Govt. Sheep Breeding and Research Farms	6 Nos
1. S.B.F. Reasi	
2. S.B.F. Billawar	
3. S.B.F. Panthal	
4. S.B.F. Balnoi	
5. S.B.F. Thathri	
6. S.B.F. Chanderkote (by internal arrangement)	
Govt. Goat Farms	1 No
1. Dairy Goat Farm Rajbagh	
Govt. Fodder Development Farms	1 No
1. Fodder Development Farm Lam	
Divisional Disease Investigation Laboratory	1 No

Dependent population

Number of rural households and household enterprises in Jammu and Kashmir having sheep and goat is 2.6 Lakhs and 2.3 Lakhs, respectively. Whereas the same number in urban areas is about 10 thousand for sheep and 6 thousand goats (Livestock Census, 2012).

Scenario of Import and export of small ruminant in J&K

S.No	Division	Sheep & Goat Population (in Lakhs)	Mutton/ Chevon Production (in Lakh Kg.)	Import of Mutton (in Lakh Kg.)	Total Mutton Availability (in Lakh Kg.)	Human Population (in Lakhs)	Non-Veg. Population (in Lakhs)
1	Jammu	39.07	169.20	63.00	232.20	44.30	26.58
2	Kashmir	21.68	106.88	147.00	253.88	54.77	54.77
3	Ladakh	6.39	24.54	0.00	24.54	2.91	2.91
	Total	**67.14**	**300.62**	**210.00**	**510.62**	**101.98**	**84.26**

a) 70% of wool exported to neighbouring states for apparel industry.

b) State meets 45% of annual local mutton requirements at present.

Mutton requirements

Total requirement of mutton @ 35 gram per day per person for 313 days (ICMR Recommendations) for given human population = 1121.78 Lakh Kg

Requirement for Non-vegetarian population = 926.86 Lakh Kg

Mutton availability

Local source	=	300.62 Lakh Kg
Imports	=	210.00 Lakh Kg
Total mutton availability	=	510.62 Lakh Kg

Mutton deficit

Whole population	=	611.16 Lakh Kg
Non-Veg. Population	=	416.24 Lakh Kg

Area covered

All districts of Jammu and Kashmir and prime areas are Srinagar, Shopian, Pulwama, Leh, Kupwara, Kulgam, Ganderbal, Budgam, Bandipora, Baramulla and Anantnag in Kashmir province, where as from Jammu the Prime areas are Kathua, Kishtwar, Rajouri, Poonch, Reasi and Udhampur.

Institutional arrangements

The institutional arrangements under the department are as:

i) **Directorate of Animal Husbandry Jammu/Kashmir:** Responsible for carrying the mandate for all the livestock except small ruminants. Each Directorate is headed by a Director Animal Husbandry.

ii) **Department of Sheep Husbandry Jammu/Kashmir:** Dedicated for development of small ruminants and Rabbits. Each Directorate is headed by a Director Sheep Husbandry.

iii) **Livestock Development Boards, Jammu / Kashmir:** Apex body to carry out the mandate of Genetic upgradation under NPCBB a Centrally Sponsored Scheme. Each Livestock Development Board is headed by a CEO.

iv) **J & K Sheep & Sheep Products Development Board, J&K:** This is headed by a Managing Director.

Breeds of Small Ruminants suitable for rearing in J&K

Breeds of Sheep: Gurezi, Gaddi, Karnahi, Bakerwali, Changthangi, Poonchi, Kashmir Merino, Corriedale, Dorper, Rambouillet

Breeds of Goat: Pashmina, Chegu, Jamunapari, Beetal, Barbari.

Exotic Breeds: The principal exotic dairy breeds of goats are Toggenberg, Sannen, French Alpine and Nubian. They are all noted for their higher milk yield and most of these breed, were imported to India to improve milk yield of our local breeds and to upgrade our non descript goats.

Small Ruminant Husbandry in J&K

a) The State is blessed with land, environment and socio-cultural setup uniquely appropriate for production of small ruminant production. The Sheep & Goat rearing in the State is the prime occupation of many rural households and tribes.

b) While the sheep population experienced around 8% growth between 2003 and 2007, the goats grew only by 0.4%. The main contribution of this sub-sector is in much demand for fine wool and mutton. To fully exploit this potential, the J&K State has established an independent Directorate for Sheep Husbandry.

c) Kashmir Merino, Gurezi and Karnah are the important sheep breeds in Kashmir, while as Rambouillet, Bakerwal cross, Punchi, Kagani and Beetal are the dominant sheep and goat breeds in Jammu. Around 60% of the sheep are crosses with improved fine wool traits. In the cold arid region of Leh and Kargil, the production system is intensive with unique livestock viz. Pashmina goat, and Changthangi sheep.

d) Breeding Sheep for Quality Wool Production: Merino and Rambouillet fine Wool breeds have been used to upgrade local sheep since early 1960s. As a result, Kashmir Merino breed was evolved. The wool quality of Kashmir Merino is comparable to the best wool in the world.

e) As of now, 70% sheep have been upgraded and have desired quality wool. Wool production during 10th plan grew by 36%. Due to minuscule A.I programme in Sheep and Goat and limited availability of breeding rams, inbreeding is on the rise.

f) Breeding Sheep for Mutton production over the 10th plan witnessed much lower growth than wool production (26% v/s 36%). Selective breeding of sheep for better and more wool has been the emphasis in the past in spite of the fact that there were adequate returns from mutton in comparison to wool.

g) The Department has started a pilot study on embryo transfer technology (ETT) programme wherein surrogate ewes have been implanted with imported embryos of exotic sheep viz. Dorper, Corridale and Rambouillet. Although the current exercise yielded only 8% lambs, importation of more embryos after proper training of the staff performance, acclimatization and survivability under existing agro climatic condition is under consideration.

h) Goat Breeding is an integral part of most of the sheep rearers in the state. The Gujjar and Bakerwals tribes usually cherish rearing of goats, thereby augmenting the income of the poorest of poor community of the state. Goat milk is used at home and the animals are sold for meat. The unfavourable conditions in the state resulting in restricting of grazing areas, Lack of effective breeding policy and Lack of goat Development programmes in the state, and haphazard slaughter of goats to meet the ever increasing demand for meat are some of the causes of subdued goat production in the state.

i) Goat population in J&K (20.63 Lakhs) remained almost stagnant since 2003. No effective goat development programme is operational at the moment although introduction of Beetal and Boer breeds of goat, and conservation of Kagani goat have been started in collaboration with SKUAST, particularly in respect of Boer goat at Bandipora Kashmir.

Small ruminant development programmes

Centrally Sponsored Schemes under Operation

1. **Assistance to States for Control of Animal Diseases (ASCAD)**

The scheme is funded by Department of Animal Husbandry, Dairying & Fisheries, Government of India on 75:25 basis (75% Central Share and 25% State Share). Following Components are taken up under the Scheme:

- Vaccination against Foot and Mouth Disease (FMD), Peste Des Petits ruminants (PPR), Sheep Pox (SP) and Clostridial infestations.
- Strengthening of Disease Diagnostic Laboratories.
- Training Programme for Veterinarians and Para Vets.
- Organization of District/ Block level Awareness Camps for breeders.
- Monitoring and Surveillance.

2. Rashtrya Krishi Vikas Yojna (RKVY)

The scheme is funded by Ministry of Agriculture & Cooperation, Department of Animal Husbandry, Dairying & Fisheries, Government of India (100% Centrally Sponsored).

Salient features of the Scheme are

- Genetic Up-gradation of sheep and goats by providing quality Germplasm to the breeders.
- Employment generation through organized sheep and goat farming on participatory mode and Machine Shearing cum Training Programme.
- Strengthening/Creation of infrastructure including establishment of polyclinics, purchase of camp equipments, solar lanterns, tractors for farms, etc.
- New Initiatives for skill development by organizing study tours of farmers.
- Increased fodder production by providing fodder seed mini-kits.

3. Integrated Sample Survey (ISS)

The scheme is funded by Department of Animal Husbandry, Dairying & Fisheries, Government of India on 50:50 basis (50% Central Share and 50% State Share). This Scheme has been taken up by Sheep Husbandry Department Jammu in Poonch, Rajouri and Kathua districts of Jammu Division. Under the scheme, estimation of livestock and livestock products on yearly basis is being conducted by staff of the Department.

4. Integrated Development of Small Ruminants and Rabbits (IDSRR)

The scheme is funded by Ministry of Agriculture & Cooperation, Department of Animal Husbandry, Dairying & Fisheries, Government of India (100% Centrally Sponsored). The scheme is being implemented in State w.e.f. 2010-11 onwards. The salient features of the Scheme are:

- Creation of Venture Capital Fund to foster area/ cluster based integrated Development as a viable commercial activity.
- Strengthening of infrastructure, human resource, institutions and rearers' organizations for rapid improvement of these species.
- Developing a skill pool of NGOs for taking up development projects on PPP mode.
- Resource mapping in identified districts for sheep, goat & rabbit in terms of raw material source as well as consumption pattern and potential.

Schemes Undertaken under IDSRR

1. **Revival of Potential Farms:**
   - Strengthening of Sheep Breeding Farm- Proposal for strengthening of SBF Reasi.
2. **Innovative Projects:**
   - Project Proposals for Embryo Transfer Technology to be implemented jointly by Sheep Husbandry Department & SKUAST-J.
3. **Organized Sheep and Goat Farming (Credit linked, funding through NABARD):**
   - Scheme to be implemented during remaining period of 11th FYP in all districts of State.

- Beneficiaries shall be SHGs, individuals, unemployed youth, preference to women, SCs and STs.
- NGOs selected by NABARD shall identify beneficiaries; act as facilitators for training of beneficiaries and sponsorship of cases to banks.
- Provision of Sheep/ Goat rearing units of 25 ewes/ does + 1 ram/ buck at estimated cost of Rs. 1.00 lacs where backend subsidy of 33.33% shall be provided & margin money 10% (Rs. 0.10 lac) shall be arranged by beneficiary & Rs. 0.90 lac shall be Bank Loan.
- Provision of Sheep/ Goat breeding farms of 500 ewes/ does + 25 rams/ bucks at estimated cost of Rs. 25.00 lacs where backend subsidy of 33.33% shall be provided & margin money 25% (Rs. 6.25 lac) shall be arranged by beneficiary & Rs. 18.75 lac shall be Bank Loan.

4. **Rural Infrastructure Development Fund.**
5. **Establishment and Strengthening of Veterinary Hospitals and Dispensaries (ESVHD) under Livestock Health and Disease Control Programme (LH&DC).**

Employment Generation Schemes in Sheep Husbandry Sector

A. State Sector Mini Sheep Farm Scheme (50 Ewes+ 2 Rams)

Particulars	Description
Sponsored by	State Government
Description	Establishment of credit linked Mini Sheep Farms of 50 Ewes and 2 Rams at cost of Rs. 2.38 lacs for unemployed youth of State. Margin Money of Rs. 0.38 lacs to be borne by beneficiary. · Rs. 2.00 lacs credit through J&K Bank Backend subsidy of Rs. 0.60 lacs to be paid by Sheep Husbandry Department to concerned branch of J&K Bank. Employment Generation for two persons on establishment of unit.
Beneficiaries	Small marginal farmers, Agriculture labourers, entrepreneurs and unemployed youth of State.

Benefit type	Rs. 0.60 lacs back ended subsidy
Eligibility criteria	Possession of minimum wherewithal viz. land, grazing rights, etc. Experience/ knowledge of trade Willingness to undergo mandatory training in management, recordkeeping etc. Willingness to invest margin money.
How to avail	Interested beneficiaries to apply to concerned District Sheep Husbandry Officers. Selection of beneficiaries by committee under Chairmanship of Additional District Development Commissioner.

B. Establishment of 25 ewes/does units on participatory mode -Centrally Sponsored – Rashtrya Krishi Vikas Yojna (RKVY)

Particulars	Description
Sponsored by	Government of India (CSS)
Description	Establishment of Sheep and Goat units of 25 ewes and 1 ram & 25 does + 1 buck at a cost of Rs 1.00 lac for unemployed youth of Jammu division. Unit to be provided on loan under participatory mode, wherein from third year onwards, 5 Ewes/ Does shall be retrieved from the beneficiary for subsequent 5 years. Retrieved livestock shall be utilized for establishment of further units. Employment Generation for one person on establishment of unit.
Beneficiaries	Small marginal farmers/ unemployed youth of State.
Benefit type	25 Ewes/ Does to be provided to beneficiaries on loan which shall be retrieved from beneficiaries in subsequent years.
Eligibility criteria	Possession of minimum wherewithal viz. land, grazing rights, etc. Experience/ knowledge of trade

	Willingness for retrieval of livestock in 5 years starting from 3rd year onwards on affidavit duly attested by First Class Magistrate.
How to avail	Interested beneficiaries to apply to concerned District Sheep Husbandry Officers.
	Selection by DSHOs and BVOs of concerned areas.

C. Establishment of Sheep/Goat units of 25 ewes/does + 1ram/buck rearing units & 500 ewes/ does + 25 Rams/ Bucks breeding units under Centrally Sponsored – Integrated Development of Small Ruminants and Rabbits (IDSRR)

Particulars	Description
Sponsored by	Government of India (CSS).
Description	Scheme to be implemented in all districts of State. · Identification of beneficiaries by identified NGOs/ Department.
	Training of the beneficiaries in organized sheep and goat rearing.
	Establishment of Credit linked Sheep/ goat rearing units of 25 ewes/ does & 1 ram/ buck at a cost of Rs. 1.00 lacs for unemployed youth of State. · Establishment of Credit linked Sheep/ goat breeding units of 500 ewes/ does & 25 rams/ bucks at a cost of Rs. 25.00 lacs for unemployed youth of State.
	Margin money 10% & 25% for rearing and breeding units respectively to be born by beneficiary.
	Rs. 0.90 lac & 18.75 lacs credit/ loan through identified Banks for rearing and breeding units respectively.
	Back-end subsidy of 33.33% to be extended by NABARD to concerned branches of Banks.
Beneficiaries	Individual farmers, Self Help Groups (SHGs) for rearing units. Preference for traditional shepherds, women, SCs and STs.
	Individual farmers, NGOs, entrepreneurs for breeding units.
Benefit type	33.3% Back ended subsidy to be extended by NABARD.

Eligibility criteria	Possession of minimum wherewithal viz. land, grazing rights, etc. Experience/ knowledge of trade · Willingness to undergo mandatory training in management, record keeping etc. Willingness to invest margin money.
How to avail	Interested beneficiaries to apply to concerned NGOs/ District Sheep Husbandry Officers. Selection by NGOs/ Service area banks. Sanction of cases by SLSMC headed by Commissioner Secretary to Government Animal/ Sheep Husbandry Department, J&K.

Economics for small scale small ruminant farming

Economics of Goat Rearing
(60+3 – One year – Stall Feeding System) (For meat purpose)

I Assumptions

1) Cost of a buck and one doe is taken at Rs. 5500 and Rs. 4500 respectively.
2) Animal will be reared under stall feeding system.
3) Animals require 15 sq.ft/ buck, 10 sq.ft/ doe and 4 sq. ft / kid of floor area and construction cost of shed is taken at Rs. 200/ sq. ft.
4) Cost of equipment is taken at Rs. 200/ goat.
5) Depreciation on building and equipment is taken at 20 % per annum.
6) Animals will be insured at the premium rate of 6% of value of animals.
7) Bucks will be fed with 200 gm of concentrate per day for 5 months and 4 kg of green fodder daily. Doe will be fed with 200 gm per day for 5 months and 4 Kg of Green fodder daily and kids with 100 gm of concentrate per day and 2 kg of green fodder daily for 5 months.
8) The cost of 1 Kg of concentrate is taken at the rate of Rs 20 and green fodder @ Rs 3/Kg.
9) The family labour (Male/Female) will be employed.
10) Veterinary expenses will be taken at Rs. 200 / goat / year and Rs. 100 / kid / year.
11) In total , 120 kids will be obtained and they will be sold at the rate of Rs. 4000/ kid (at 9 months of age)

II	**Fixed Investment**		**Rs.**
	1 Cost of 3 Bucks @ Rs. 5500 each		16500/-
	2 Cost of 60 does @ Rs. 4500 each		270000/-
	3 Cost of building 100 kids x 4 sq.ft/ kid60x 10sq.ft/ doe and 3 x 15 sq.ft/ buck @ Rs. 200 / sq.ft.		209000/-
	4 Cost of equipment @ Rs. 200/adult goat		12600/-
	Total Fixed Investment		**508100/-**
III	**Fixed Cost**		
	1 Interest on fixed investment @ 15% annum		76215/-
	2 Depreciation of building @ 10% /annum		20900/-
	3 Deprecation on equipment @ 20% /annum		2520/-
	4 Insurance charges @ 6% of value of animals		17190/-
	Total Fixed Cost		**116825/-**
IV	**Variable Cost**		
	1 **Cost of concentrate**		
	200 gm /day /buck for 2 months(36 Kgs)	3636 kgs x	72720/-
	200 gm /day/doe for 5 months(1800 Kgs)	Rs.20	
	100 gm / day/ kid for 5 months (1800 Kgs)		
	Cost of green fodder		
	4 Kg/ day/buck for 365 days (4380 Kg)	127980 Kgs x	255960/-
	4 Kg/ day/doe for 365 days (87600 Kg)	Rs 2	
	2 Kg/ day/Kid for 5 months (36000 Kg)		
	2 Veterinary charge @ Rs. 200/Year/goat @ 100 /year/kid		24600/-
	Total Variable cost		**353280/-**
V	**Total cost (III +IV)**		**470105/-**
VI	**Returns**		
	1 By sale of kids @ Rs.4500/each x 120 kids		540000/-
	2 Sale of manure		60000 /-
	3 By sale of empty gunny bag		1250
	Total Returns		**601250/-**
	Net Returns per year (VI - V)		**131145/-**
	Net Returns per month		**10928.75/-**

Economics of Sheep Unit
(20+1 – Two years) for meat purpose

1	**Assumptions**	
	1 Cost of a ram is taken at Rs 5500 and cost of a ewe is taken at Rs. 4500.	
	2 Cost of construction of a kutcha pen is taken at 45000 and equipment worth of Rs. 5000 will be bought.	
	3 Depreciation on building and equipment is taken at 20% per annum.	
	4 Animals will be insured at a premium rate of 6% of value of animals.	
	5 As animals will be reared under extensive system, veterinary charges alone are accounted. Veterinary charges are taken at Rs. 200 / Animal / year.	
	6 The family labour (Male/ Female) will be employed.	
	7 Apart from grazing Ram is fed with 200g concentrate feed per day for one month, ewe with 200g/ day for 6 months and lambs with 100g/day for 3 months & cost of 1 Kg of Concentrate feed is taken @ Rs 20/ Kg	
	8 In total 32 lambs will be obtained in two years (16 lambs in each lambing, lambs will be sold at Rs. 4500 / lamb at 9 months of age).	
II	**Fixed Investment**	**Rs.**
	1 Cost of one ram	5500/-
	2 Cost of 20 ewes @ Rs. 4500	90000/-
	3 Cost of construction of a kutcha pen	45000
	4 Cost of equipment	5000
	Total Fixed Investment	**145500/-**
III	**Fixed cost**	
	1 Interest on fixed investment @ 15%/annum	21825/-
	2 Depreciation on pen and equipment @ 20%/annum	10000/-
	3 Insurance cost @ 6% of value of animal/annum	5730/-
	Total Fixed cost (for 2 yrs)	**37555/-**
IV	**Variable cost**	
	1 Veterinary charges @ Rs. 200/animal/year	8400/-
	2 **Cost of concentrate**	34800/-
	200gm/day/ram for 1 month (6 kg/year)	
	200gm/day/ewe for 6 month (720 kg/year)	

	100gm/day/lamb for 3 months (144 kg/ year)	
	(870 kgs x 2= 1740 kg x Rs 20)	
	Total Variable cost	**43200/-**
V	**Total cost (III +IV)**	**80755/-**
VI	**Returns**	
	1 Sale of 32 lambs @ Rs 4500 / lamb	144000/-
	2 Sale of manure	7500/-
	Total Returns	**151500/-**
	Net Returns for two years (VI – V)	**70745/-**
	Net Return per year	**35372.50/-**

8

Diagnoses of Parasitic Diseases in Livestock

M. Rashid and A. Yadav

Associate Professor, Faculty of Veterinary Sciences & Animal Husbandry SKUAST-Jammu-181102

Collection of faecal samples: To diagnose gastro-intestinal parasites of ruminants or other animals, the parasites or their eggs/larvae must be recovered from the digestive tract of animal or human or from the faecal/ stool material.

The faecal samples for parasitological examination should be collected from the rectum of animals. If rectum samples cannot be obtained, fresh faecal samples may be collected from the pastures. Several samples should be collected and immediately dispatched to the diagnostic laboratory in suitable containers such as:

- Plastic containers with lids
- Screw caped bottles
- Disposable plastic sleeves
- Plastic bags
- Gloves used for collecting the samples

Instructions

1. Each sample collected should be properly labeled with animal identification, date and place of collection.
2. Samples should be packed and dispatched in a cool box (Sample carrier) to avoid the eggs developing and hatching.
3. In long journeys where transportation takes much time fill the container to the capacity or air tighten the sleeve or plastic bag to exclude air from the container.

4. Add 3% formalin to the sample (5-20 ml. depending on the volume of sample) to preserve parasitic eggs.
5. On receiving the samples in laboratory store in refrigerator at 4°C until they are processed
6. Samples can be kept in refrigerator for upto 3 weeks without significant changes in the egg counts and the morphology of eggs.
7. Samples should never be kept in freezer.

Basic limitations of faecal examination in diagnoses of gastrointestinal parasites

1. Failure to demonstrate the parasitic eggs or larvae does not mean absence of parasites, they are present in an immature stage or the test used may not be sufficiently sensitive.
2. The demonstration of parasitic eggs or larvae in the faeces provides positive evidence but does not indicate degree of infection.
3. There is a correlation between the number of eggs/larvae per gram of faeces and the number of adult nematodes present in sheep and goats but not in cattle in mixed infection.

Factors that limit the accuracy and significance of a faecal egg count

1. There is fairly regular fluctuation in faecal egg output.
2. Eggs are not evenly distributed throughout the faeces.
3. Quantity of feaces passed will effect the number of eggs per unit weight.
4. The egg output is influenced by the season of year as more in rainy season.
5. The resistance of the host can depress or entirely inhibit the egg production of parasites.
6. Immature worms do not evidence their presence by producing eggs.
7. Eggs sometime may not be detected due to low numbers or low sensitivity of test.
8. Immunity may results in prepatent period and there by reduction in eggs production.

Faecal examination by direct smears

A small quantity of faeces placed on slide is mixed with a drop of water, spread out and then covered with a glass cover slip and examined directly using 10 X objective for parasitic eggs and larvae, 40 X for motile protozoa organisms.

Another technique of examining the faecal material is preparation of emulsion of small quantity of dung in water or normal saline and filtering through double layer of muslin cloth. Take a drop of emulsion on a glass slide, prepare smear, cover with cover slip and examined directly using 10X objective for parasitic eggs and larvae and 40 X for motile protozoa.

Quantitative techniques for separating and concentrating eggs/ larvae

1. Simple test tube floatation
2. Simple floatation
3. Sedimentation technique for trematode eggs
4. Microscopic examination of prepared samples.

A number of different methods are available for separation, concentration and demonstration of eggs, oocysts and larvae in faecal samples. The 3 methods described are as:

1. Simple test tube floatation
2. Simple floatation method
3. Sedimentation technique for trematode eggs.

Simple test tube floatation

Principle

The simple test tube floatation method is a qualitative test for the detection of nematodes and cestode eggs and coccidian oocysts in the faeces. It is based on the separation of eggs from faecal material and concentrating them by means of a floatation fluid with an appropriate specific gravity.

Application

It is good technique to be used for initial survey to establish the group of parasites.

Procedures

1. Weigh 3 gms of faeces/stool sample in a container.
2. Pour 50 ml. of floatation fluid into container.
3. Mix thoroughly.
4. Filter the resulting faecal suspension through a strainer or a double layer of cheese cloth.
5. Pour the faecal suspension into a test tube from container.
6. Place test tube in a test tube stand or rack.
7. Gently top up the test tube with faecal suspension leaving a convex meniscus at the top of the tube and carefully place a cover slip over it.
8. Allow the test tube to stand for 20 minutes.
9. Remove the cover slip carefully with a drop of fluid adhere to it and examined by placing on a clean glass slide under the microscope.

Simple floatation method

Principle

Principle is same as that of simple test tube floatation method.

Application

This is another good technique for use in initial surveys. It can be useful in detecting low numbers of eggs along with MacMaster Technique.

Procedure

1. Take 3 gms of faeces into a container 1.
2. Emulsify with 50 ml. of floatation fluid.
3. Filter the resulting faecal suspension through a strainer or a double layer of cheese cloth.

4. Pour the faecal suspension into another container from container 1.
5. Place the container 2 to stand for 10 minutes.
6. Press a test tube to the bottom of the filtrate, lift it quickly and transfer a few drops adhering to the surface to a glass slide.
7. Allow the test tube to touch the slide for 2-4 seconds for the drops to run off.
8. Mount the cover slip on a clean glass slide and examine under the microscope.

Sedimentation technique for trematode eggs

Principle

The sedimentation technique is a qualitative method for detecting trematode eggs (*Paraamphistomum*) in the faeces. Most trematode eggs are relatively large and heavy as compared to nematode eggs. This technique concentrates them in sediment.

Procedure

1. Weigh approximately 3 g of faeces into a container 1.
2. Emulsify it with 40-50 ml tape water.
3. Mix thoroughly with a stirring device.
4. Filter the resulting faecal suspension through a strainer or a double layer of cheese cloth, into a container 2.
5. Pour the faecal suspension into a test tube from container 2.
6. Allow the sediment for 5 minutes.
7. Remove the supernatant very carefully.
8. Re-suspend the sediment in 5 ml. of water.
9. Allow the sediment for 5 minutes.
10. Discard the supernatant very carefully.
11. Stain the sediment by adding one drop of methylene blue.
12. Transfer the sediment to a microslide and cover with a coverslip.

Microscopic examination of prepared samples

The prepared samples on microslides from the simple test tube flotation method, simple flotation method and sedimentation method are examined under a microscope at the magnifications listed in Table below:

Table: Magnification levels for examining prepared samples

Magnification	Parasites
10×10	Nematode and cestode eggs
10×40	Coccidian oocysts
10×4	Trematodes

Warning: In case of a time delay between processing the sample and reading the count, egg numbers may decline dramatically. Also the eggs may change their appearance, becoming crenated and "gost-like". It is therefore advisable to prepare only a few samples at a time. These changes can be prevented by keeping prepared samples in the refrigerator after mixing. Using the salt sugar solution as flotation fluid also reduces the morphological changes.

Quantitative Techniques for separating and concentrating eggs/ larvae

The simplest and the most effective method for determining the number of eggs or oocysts per gram of faeces is the McMaster counting technique described below:

McMaster counting technique

Principle

The McMaster counting technique is a quantitative technique to determine the number of eggs present per gram of faeces. A floatation fluid is used to separate eggs from faecal material in a counting chamber (McMaster) with two compartments. The technique described below will detect 50 or more egg per gm. of faeces.

The technique is used to quantify the eggs of nematodes, cestodes and coccidian.

Procedure

1. Take 4 gm of sample into a container 1.
2. Add 56 ml. of floatation fluid.
3. Mix and emulsify thoroughly with a stirring device.
4. Filter the resulting faecal suspension through a strainer or a double layer of cheese cloth.
5. While straining into container 2, take a sub-sample with a Pasteur pipette.
6. Fill both side of the McMaster chamber with the sub-sample.
7. Allow counting chamber to stand for 5 minutes (important).
8. Examine the sub-sample of filtrate under microscope at 10×10 magnification.
9. Count all eggs & coccidian oocysts within engraved area of both chambers (MacMaster).
10. The number of the eggs per gm. of faeces can be calculated as follows:

Example: Add the egg counts of the two chambers together. Multiply the total by 50. This is the egg count per gm of faeces. For example if we have counted 10 eggs in chamber 1 and 15 eggs in chamber 2. Total eggs are= 10+15= 25, so eggs per gm of faeces will be 25×50=1250.

Note: in case we did not got any egg or oocyst in the MacMaster chamber, the filtrate in the container can be used for simple floatation method by taking the steps as:

a) Press a test tube to the bottom of the filtrate, lift it quickly and transfer a few drops adhering to the surface to a glass slide.
b) Allow the test tube to touch the slide for 2-4 seconds for the drops to run off.
c) Mount the cover slip on slide and examine under the microscope.

Warning: In case of a time delay between processing the sample and reading the count, egg numbers may decline dramatically. Also the eggs may change their appearance, becoming crenated and "gost-like". It is therefore advisable to prepare only a few samples at a time. These changes can be prevented by keeping prepared samples in the refrigerator after mixing. Using the salt sugar solution as flotation fluid also reduces the morphological changes.

Guidelines for interpretation of faecal egg counts in young animals

The degree of eggs per gm of faeces in different species are expressed as below in the Table.

Table –faecal egg counts per gm in young animals

Parasite	Degree of infection (epg) of faeces		
Cattle	**Light**	**Moderate**	**Heavy**
Mixed infection	50-200	200-800	800+
Pure *Haemonchus* infection	200	200-600	600+
Pure *Trichostrongylus* infection	50-100	100-400	400+
Pure *Cooperia* infection	200-300	300-2500	2500+
Sheep			
Mixed infection	50-800	800-1200	1200+
Mixed infection with *Haemonchus*	300-800	800-1000	1000+
Pure *Haemonchus* infection	100-2000	2000-7000	7000+
Pure *Trichostrongylus* infection	100-500	500-2000	2000+
Pure *Nematodirus* infection	50-100	100-600	600+
Pure *Oesophagostomum*	100-800	800-1600	1600+

The guidelines should be established on research bases under different climatic condition in different areas depending upon the number of parasites their impact of pathogens on the livestock etc. but this is a rough idea established by some other scientist for hot humid climate.

Identification of mite

Skin scrapings that contain dead mites, large amounts of skin flakes or scabs or large amounts of hair processed further as:

1. Place the skin scraping (up to several grams of skin and hair) in a suitable size beaker, then add sufficient 10% potassium hydroxide to immerse the sample.
2. Cautiously bring the solution to a gentle boil, stirring frequently (a laboratory hot-plate with a magnetic stirrer works well for this), for 5–10 minutes or long enough to digest most of the hair and skin. This step will be performed under a chemical fume hood to limit exposure to caustic fumes.
3. Avoid boiling for an extended period of time so that the mites may not disintegrate. Transfer the digested material to suitable test tubes and centrifuge at 600 *g* for 10 minutes.
4. Decant the supernatant.
5. Re-suspended the pellet in a small amount of flotation medium (e.g. Sheather's solution); then, fill the tube completely with flotation medium and place a cover slip on top of the tube, assuring that it makes contact with the flotation medium.
6. Allow to stand for 1 hour, or centrifuged for 10 minutes.
7. Carefully remove the cover slip by lifting straight up, so that a drop of fluid remains on the underside of the cover slip and place on a glass slide.
8. Any mites in the sample will float to the top and will be found in the drop of fluid attached to the cover slip. Another simpler but satisfactory technique, that is used is re-suspension of the pellet in a small amount of distilled water, drop onto a large (76 × 51 × 1 mm) glass slide and covered with a 40 × 50 mm cover-slip.
9. This will be examined under a dissecting microscope (×40 or ×100) with under stage lighting.
10. The slide then be examined under a compound microscope for the presence of mites.

Laboratory diagnosis of protozoan infections

For identification of trophozoites and cysts of the intestinal amoebae, flagellates and ciliates permanently stained faecal smears are prepared. Trophozoite stages are most often found in watery or diarrhoeic faecal specimens in severe cases where usually cysts are not seen in such specimens. On the other hand, cysts are the stage typically found in formed faecal specimens. A mixture of trophozoites and cysts may occur in softer and semi-formed faeces.

In direct smears of faeces in saline, motile trophozoites may be found. A motile amoebic trophozoite containing red blood cells is immediately identifiable as *E. histolytica*. Motile amoebic trophozoites that do not contain ingested erythrocytes are more difficult to classify and are best diagnosed in permanently stained smears. However, experienced technicians can often identify species accurately in wet mount faecal preparations, but permanently stained smears are superior to saline- or iodine-stained wet mounts.

Oocysts of the intestinal coccidians can be identified in wet mount faecal preparations, principally on the basis of size or shape. They typically do not stain well with trichrome or iron haematoxylin. The use of acid-fast staining of faecal smears is superior for demonstrating these oocysts. The extremely small size of microsporidian spores makes their identification difficult under any circumstance.

Modification of the trichrome stain by increasing the amount of the stain components and increasing the time for staining aids in demonstrating the spores in faeces.

Flotation and sedimentation faecal concentration procedures are not useful for demonstrating trophozoite stages of the intestinal protozoa but can be highly efficient for demonstrating cyst stages.

Permanent stains for faecal smears

Trichrome stain

Use: Very good stain for fresh and PVA (polyvinyl alcohol fixative) preserved faecal smears: does not give good staining results with SAF (sodium acetate, acetic acid, formalin) preservation.

Preparation: Add 10 ml of glacial acetic acid to 6 g of chromotrope 2R, 3 g of light green SF and 7 g of phosphotungstic acid in a clean flask. Swirl to mix and let stand for 30 min. Add 1000 ml of distilled water and mix thoroughly; the stain should be a deep purple. Store in a glass-stoppered bottle; the stain is stable and is used undiluted.

Staining procedure: Place slides, fixed in either Schaudinn's fixative or PVA, into 70% alcohol for 2 min. Add Lugol's diluted iodine solution to 70% ethanol to produce a colour of strong tea: place slides in the solution for 5 min. Place slides in two changes of 70% alcohol.

Stain slides in undiluted trichrome stain for 10 min. Remove slides, drain thoroughly, and place them in 90% acidified alcohol (prepared by adding 4.5 ml of glacial acetic acid to 1 litre of 90% ethanol) for 2-3 seconds. Dip slides in 95% alcohol to rinse and then dehydrate through 100% ethanol and xylene or through carbol-xylene mixture. Using resinous mounting medium, place a cover slip on the smear.

Iron haematoxylin stain

Use: Very good stain for fresh, PVA- or SAF-preserved faecal smears.

Preparation

Stock solution A: dissolve 1 g of haematoxylin crystals in 100 ml of 95% alcohol; allow solution to stand in light for 1 week and then filter.

Stock solution B: mix 1 g of ferrous ammonium sulfate, 1 g of ferric ammonium sulfate and 1 ml of hydrochloric acid in 97 ml of distilled water. Prepare a working solution by combining 25 ml each of stock solutions A and B; prepare at least 3-4 h prior to staining. Prepare picric acid solution for destaining by adding 25 ml of saturated aqueous picric acid to 25 ml of distilled water.

Staining procedure: Place slides into 70% alcohol for 5 min; into 50% alcohol for 2 min; into tap water for 5 min; into working haematoxylin stain solution for 10 min; into distilled water for 1 min; into picric acid solution for 1 min; into running tap water for 10 min; into 70% alcohol containing 1 drop of ammonia for 5 min; and into 95% alcohol for 5 min. Dehydrate through 100% ethanol and xylene or through carbol-xylene mixture. Using resinous mounting medium, place a cover slip on the smear.

Modified Ziehl-Neelsen technique (acid-fast stain)

Use: For detection of *C. parvum*, *C. cayetanensis*, and other coccidian infections.

Reagents: Carbol-fuchsin, formalin, HCl-ethanol solution, glycerol malachite green (or methylene blue) solution, HCl-methanol solution.

Staining procedure: Prepare a thin smear of faeces; air-dry and fix in methanol for 2-3 min. Stain with cold carbol-fuchsin for 5-10 min.

Differentiate in 1% HCl-ethanol until colour ceases to flow out of smear. Rinse in tapwater. Counterstain with 0.25% malachite green (or methylene blue) for 30 sec. Rinse in tapwater. Blot or drain dry.

Common floatation fluids/solutions

The common fluids/solutions in use are:

- Saturated solution of common salt (NaCl) of Sp.Gr.1.18-1.19
- Saturated sugar/sucrose solution of Sp. Gr. 1.25
- Saturated solution of sodium nitrate
- Glycerine
- Zinc sulphate solution (32.5 % solution) of Sp.Gr.1.18
- A.E.X. (Acid HCl of Sp.Gr.1.03 + Ether + Xylol equal parts)
- Magnesium sulphate.

Suggested readings

1. Wikipedia, The Free Encyclopedia.
2. Basic Laboratory Methods in Medical Parasitology by WHO 1991.
3. Training Manual on Diagnosis of Intestinal Parasites 2004.
4. Soulsby EJL (1982) Helminths, arthropods and protozoa of domesticated animals, 7th ed, Bailliere and Tindal, London, Uk.